Your Hormone Doctor

'If you are a woman, live with a woman or know a woman, this book will be your new best friend.' Emilia Fox

'Empowering for women of any age.' Lulu

Your Hormone Doctor

LEAH HARDY AND
SUSIE ROGERS
with DR DANIEL SISTER

MICHAEL JOSEPH
an imprint of
PENGUIN BOOKS

MICHAEL JOSEPH

Published by the Penguin Group

Penguin Books Ltd, 80 Strand, London WC2R ORL, England

Penguin Group (USA) Inc., 375 Hudson Street, New York, New York 10014, USA

Penguin Group (Canada), 90 Eglinton Avenue East, Suite 700, Toronto, Ontario, Canada M4P 2Y3

(a division of Pearson Penguin Canada Inc.)

Penguin Ireland, 25 St Stephen's Green, Dublin 2, Ireland (a division of Penguin Books Ltd)

Penguin Group (Australia), 707 Collins Street, Melbourne, Victoria 3008, Australia

(a division of Pearson Australia Group Pty Ltd)

Penguin Books India Pvt Ltd, 11 Community Centre, Panchsheel Park, New Delhi – 110 017, India

Penguin Group (NZ), 67 Apollo Drive, Rosedale, Auckland 0632, New Zealand

(a division of Pearson New Zealand Ltd)

Penguin Books (South Africa) (Pty) Ltd, Block D, Rosebank Office Park,

181 Jan Smuts Avenue, Parktown North, Gauteng 2193, South Africa

Penguin Books Ltd, Registered Offices: 80 Strand, London WC2R ORL, England

www.penguin.com

First published 2014

002

Set in 13.5/16 pt Garamond MT Std
Typeset by Jouve (UK), Milton Keynes

Printed in Great Britain by Clays Ltd, St Ives plc
A CIP catalogue record for this book is available from the British Library

ISBN: 978–1–405–91542–7

www.greenpenguin.co.uk

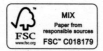

Contents

Leah Hardy

Leah Hardy is a well-known health and beauty journalist with a career that spans two decades. She began working on glossy magazines in the UK, including working as deputy editor, and then editor, of UK *Cosmopolitan*. As a freelance journalist, she developed a passionate interest in health and anti-ageing beauty, writing for most of the major newspapers, particularly the *Daily Mail, The Times* and *The Sunday Times*, and for glossy magazines including *Red, Easy Living, Harper's Bazaar, Top Santé* and *Zest*. She has appeared on radio and TV, edited a medical journal for cosmetic doctors, spoken at medical conferences and worked as a consultant for major medical companies launching in the anti-ageing market. Leah is married with two children and a grown-up stepdaughter, and lives in London.

Susie Rogers

A native New Yorker, Susie has made her home in the UK for over thirty-five years. Her early years were spent in the music business, after which she founded and taught at BodyWorksWest, the first Pilates studio in Notting Hill,

London. Given her abiding passion for beauty and well-being, in 2005 she opened BeautyWorksWest medispa with Dr Daniel Sister. With its advanced scientific beauty techniques and exceptional service, it fast became a firm favourite with the press, attracting a loyal following. In 2011, Susie and Dr Sister launched their own beauty line, including the hero product YOUTH, which was an instant, sell-out success. Susie is often featured in the press, and her views on beauty and health are much sought after. Susie has a son, daughter and granddaughter, and lives with her partner in London and Wiltshire.

Dr Daniel Sister

World-renowned anti-ageing specialist Dr Daniel Sister practises exclusively at BeautyWorksWest. He received his medical doctorate at the Paris Medical University (Broussais-Hôtel Dieu), subsequently building a global reputation. He has practised at many of the world's foremost clinics, written several highly acclaimed books, and regularly appears on TV. His extensive research studies and expert-ise are sought after by the beauty, anti-ageing, nutrition and complementary medical communities. A market leader and pioneer, he has introduced a number of groundbreaking treatments to the UK market, attracting worldwide atten-tion and featuring in both the national and medical press.

INTRODUCTION

Stop hor-moaning, and take control of your hormones, health and happiness right now

We guess you are reading this book for a reason. Maybe you've just reached an age when you've started to get curious about what's going to happen to your mind and body in the second phase of your life. Maybe you've started to notice small changes that you suspect may be linked to your hormones – your cycle isn't what it was; you don't sleep as well; you feel tired and moody. Or maybe the changes are more physical – your body is changing; you might find your weight keeps going up and you can't shift that roll of fat around the middle that's stopping you wearing half the clothes in your wardrobe. Perhaps the face in the mirror is changing in ways you didn't expect – where did those lines come from? What's happening to your jaw-line? Or perhaps it's more basic than that – you feel old; the zing has gone; your old youthful energy has faded; you don't have the same enthusiasm and positivity, let alone, ahem, the same libido. Maybe you are scared that this is your future?

Well, wake up! This isn't your destiny. Not any more. As

a woman in mid-life the world is at your feet. You *are* the future. United Nations figures show that right now, one in four women is over fifty; in five years' time, one in three will be; and in fifty years, a staggering half of all women in the world will be over fifty. And we are *not* going to be sidelined. We are absolutely refusing to retire into quiet anonymity and leave the jobs, the sex and even the rock'n'roll to the twenty-somethings. We don't act old – actor and businesswoman Jane Asher, sixty-seven, recently said, 'I'm still waiting to wake up feeling like a grown-up' – and we are not interested in looking old either. Forget the stereotypes about grey hair and cottage-loaf figures. Recently the cosmetics giant L'Oréal compiled a special report on women's attitudes to their looks, which con-cluded, 'Appearance is just as important to over fifties as under fifties.' The beauty market for fifty-plus women is estimated to be worth around £2 billion a year, and women in this age group accounted for 41 per cent of the total spend on make-up, skincare and toiletries. Women such as Elle Macpherson, fifty, Christie Brinkley, fifty-six, and Helen Mirren, sixty-six, demonstrate that age is no barrier to sexiness.

But the revolution against stereotypical ageing goes deeper than our looks. Today's mid-life woman is hard to pin down. She could be at the top of her career, as a chief executive or the editor of *Vogue*. Or she could be retired from one career and setting up a business. Many women looking at the second phase of their lives experience a sudden surge of confidence, creativity and a now-or-never determination to fulfil their ambitions. A friend of ours,

Kate Griffin, wrote her first ever novel at forty-nine, and at fifty has a major three-book publishing deal. We know mid-life women who have become yoga teachers, trained for marathons for the first time, or decided to go for the major promotion or big job they were afraid to try for before. Women in the second phase could be a grand-mother like Susie, who started her hugely successful business in mid-life, or they could still be bringing up their own young children, like Leah.

In short, for many of us, mid-life is the point when, instead of thinking of slowing down, we actually speed up, deciding to fulfil our potential. And why shouldn't we? Think of the most impressive, kick-ass women in the world, from Hillary Clinton and German chancellor Angela Merkel to Oprah Winfrey and designer Diane von Fürstenberg. Are they at the top of their game? Yup. Are they over fifty? You bet! And coming up behind them are the fabulous forty-somethings, such as J. K. Rowling and JLo, both of whom are showing no sign of slowing down. We have more opportunities in our lives, fewer restrictions and more time ahead of us, as our life spans grow ever longer. We want to make the most of this time and, thank-fully, more and more scientific evidence shows that youth – mental and physical – is something you can have at almost any age.

OK, yes, it's true you can't stop time passing. It's no good yelling at the sun for coming up every morning, or because your birthday seems to turn up every five minutes these days. But as for how time affects you? That's very different. So what do we mean by youth? For us, as women in the second phase of life – a term we use to describe women aged forty to, well, as long as they want – youth doesn't have much to do with your date of birth. Instead it's all about how healthy, fit, positive and energetic you feel; how you approach life and how you interact with other people. And, of course, how you look, too. Yes, we definitely still have our vanity. Our key message, one that we passionately believe in, is that you can take charge of the ageing process. Don't believe us? Think your hormones, your mood and your genes are just things that happen to you and that you're stuck with?

That's simply not true. The choices you make in food, drink, exercise and lifestyle – even the way you sit and stand – instantly affect your hormones. They can even change the way your genes behave.

We guess that right now you are either thinking something like, 'I'm too old to change,' or, 'Wow! This sounds interesting.' The first response will make you look older and even *be* older; the second will make you look and become younger. And that's a promise. We have the science to prove it. Follow the steps in this book and you *will* feel younger, healthier and have more energy. Your body will change; your looks will improve. Not only that, other people will notice the difference. They'll start to comment on how much younger and more positive you seem. And if they don't like it – and let's face it, plenty of people feel pretty fed up when their friends start looking and acting younger than they do – they might not pay you any compliments. But they'll definitely notice.

But before we tell you how to get younger, we are going to tell you something surprising. This may sound completely crazy, but scientists have admitted they don't know exactly what makes our bodies look and act older. There are, however, some things that they do know are part of the picture. First, there's damage caused by our lifestyles. We know stress ages the body inside and out, and the wrong food, smoking and lack of exercise are all quick ways to damage your cells and speed up the ageing process. Then there's our genetic code. It seems that to some extent you will have been born with a genetic 'ageing speed', which may be affected by our nutrition in the womb. Also, the lifespan of your cells is at least partly fixed by things called telomeres. Never heard of them? They're important. Your chromosomes exist in every cell of your body. They contain your DNA and hundreds of genes, and they are basically a set of instructions to your body. The ends of your chromosomes are capped by telomeres, which act like the plastic caps on the ends of shoelaces, protecting them and preventing them from being damaged.

Each time the cell divides to make new skin, blood, bones and other body parts, your telomeres get cut down in size a little. When the telomeres become too short, the cell commits suicide. But don't panic. Surprising new research indicates that both your 'genetic speedometer' and the length of your telomeres – and therefore the length of your cells' lives – can be affected by your lifestyle and diet. We'll tell you more about that later.

Inflammation is another cause of ageing that's attracting a

lot of attention right now. Inflammation is part of your body's immune response, but chronic inflammation can affect your entire body, and tends to get worse with age. This inflammation is deadly. It affects our cells, our hormones and contributes to ageing and chronic diseases, including diabetes, cancer and heart disease. Many doctors now believe that all so-called degenerative diseases are caused, or at least made worse, by inflammation – even Alzheimer's – and so is depression. Scary, yes, but very fixable (see Chapter 10 for how). Finally, there's hormonal ageing. As we get older, our hormones change, both in the rollercoaster ride before the menopause that's called the peri-menopause and permanently at the menopause itself. These changes are pretty dramatic and get blamed for every female ailment under the sun. And yes, those hormone changes can give you hot flushes, thin your skin, change the way your body stores fat and cause vaginal dryness (we'll definitely get back to you on that one). What this book is going to tell you, in simple and straightforward language, is what really happens during your hormone shifts.

You'll also find out how sleep, food, exercise, stress-reduction plus supplements of hormones and specific nutrients can all be used to take control of the changes in your body. In some cases, they can even reverse them. Whether you are coming up to, going through or past the menopause, you can protect your telomeres, dramatically reduce inflammation, balance your hormones, tame your hunger and rebuild lean muscle. You can actually start to get younger and healthier right this minute. And the fantastic news is that it's all easier and more fun than you might imagine. You are going to feel amazing.

Take Control!

- Ageing is not just something that happens to us, it's controlled to a surprisingly large extent by the choices we make and the lifestyles we lead. This means we can change our age destiny.
- Even the things that are inevitable, like the menopause, can affect us in different ways, depending on the choices we make and the way we think.
- Hormonal imbalances, inflammation, even the way our genes work can all be changed and improved.
- You can't stop the clock, or change your chronological age, but your real age is your biological age, and you *can* slow down and even reverse the ageing process.

'Beautiful young people are accidents of nature, but beautiful old people are works of art.'
Eleanor Roosevelt

1. Take Control: Your Hormone Connection

Look, we don't want to bore you to tears with science, science, science, but if you are a woman over forty, what's happening to your hormones is really important. Most women start to experience ups and downs as their hormones shift. Your body is extraordinary, but some of these changes can be unwelcome, so you need to understand exactly what's going on, so that you can do something about it. Oh, and we think it's really interesting, too.

It's a common mistake to think that hormones are simply responsible for your sex life and fertility, or worse, that they are just things that cause us problems, such as endometriosis, painful periods, PMT, infertility and so on. In fact, hormones are amazing. They are the source of life. They control our energy levels, the strength of our muscles and bones, and our metabolisms. Hormones send us to sleep and wake us up in the morning, make our skin bouncy, maintain our curves, our moods, memory and heart health. They keep us young, firm, strong and vital. So it's not surprising that when they decline, we end up with a lot more to deal with than just decreasing fertility.

The problem with our hormones is not that they exist, but that, as we age, they stop working in a kind of symphony, with each one playing a part to create a harmonious system. When you are young and your hormones are at

9

optimum levels, you are generally healthy, energetic and strong. But as you enter your forties and your hormones shift and decline, you can become more vulnerable to the changes and diseases associated with ageing.

We promise there are solutions to the problems caused by these natural hormonal changes, though, and before we talk about what they are, let's find out a bit more about what hormones are, and what they do.

Your body has three different communication systems – your nervous system, the endocrine system and the immune system – and each of these uses a particular type of chemical messenger. Nerve cells communicate through neurotransmitters, the endocrine system through hormones and the immune system through cytokines, and all three work together.

So let's explain in a little more depth. Hormones are chemical compounds that act, in essence, as fuel for your bodily functions. They are made by your endocrine glands, which include the pituitary gland at the base of the neck; the thyroid gland in the neck; the pancreas, which is part of the digestive system; the adrenals, which sit on top of your kidneys; and the ovaries, which sit on either side of the womb. All the hormones are then carried in your bloodstream to other organs and glands. There are receptors, or 'docking stations', for hormones all over your body and in your brain, too. When hormones lock onto their target, they stimulate that part of your body to function more vigorously or slow it down. The levels of your hormones fluctuate daily. The sex hormones, oestrogen and testosterone, are secreted in short bursts, which vary from hour to hour and even minute to minute. Hormone release also varies between night and day and from one stage of the menstrual cycle to another, in a kind of highly organ-ized 'hormone clock'. But when your hormones are balanced overall, your body is able to do miraculous things, such as generate new tissue, create an abundance of energy and fight disease.

Your Key Hormones Explained

Oestrogen

This most feminine of hormones is made primarily in the ovaries pre-menopause and, in much smaller quantities, by your adrenal glands and fat cells after the menopause. Together with progesterone, oestrogen controls your monthly cycle. What you might not know is that oestrogen is actually three hormones: oestradiol, which is the most powerful, plus oestrone and oestriol.

Oestradiol is the primary sex hormone of your young adult years. Produced mainly by the ovaries, though also by the brain, it is responsible for female physical characteristics – tits and hips, baby! – sexual functioning and fertility. It also plays a vital role in preventing middle-aged spread by driving fat to the hips and thighs and away from the waist, and is extremely important for brain function, sleep and bone health. On the down side, oestradiol also contributes to most gynaecological problems, such as endometriosis, fibroids and cancers.

Oestrone is produced by your ovaries as well as by body fat and the adrenal glands, and it is the major type of oestrogen hormone produced in any quantities once you are post-menopausal.

Oestriol is the 'weakest' form of oestrogen, and is produced by the placenta during pregnancy. But this weakness may be an advantage, in that it can be given to menopausal women as a supplement to relieve menopausal symptoms without increasing hormone-dependent cancers.

When levels of total oestrogens fall at menopause, as the ovaries stop producing the hormones, results can include thinning, dry and wrinkled skin, thinning bones, hot flushes, hair loss, urine infections, tiredness, changes in body-fat distribution, mood swings and insomnia. Older women have the same or even a greater risk of heart disease to that of men, making if the second most common killer of women in the UK, after dementia and Alzheimer's. This appears to be linked to oestrogen deficiency. Lack of oestrogen also kills off the brain's receptors for the 'reward and pleasure' chemical called dopamine, which can make it harder to concentrate and focus. You'll find out more about balancing and supplementing oestrogen further on.

Progesterone

Known as the 'calming hormone', progesterone is produced by the ovaries, the placenta during pregnancy and also by the adrenal glands.

Progesterone affects the body by increasing your metabolic rate, lowering insulin levels and enhancing thyroid hormone effects, thus boosting your metabolism. Progesterone also works as a brain hormone, boosting your brain's levels of the 'happy chemicals' dopamine and serotonin. It is also used to make the stress-controlling chemical cortisol. Healthy levels of progesterone relieve insomnia, reduce stress and depression and help the body eliminate excess body fluid. Low levels can cause anxiety, aggression, poor sleep, weight gain, bloating and water retention, and may also mean your thyroid gland cannot work properly.

Levels of progesterone start to fall about ten years before oestrogen levels do, and this has been associated with weight gain and anxiety.

Testosterone

You may think this is one that's just for the guys, but you need testosterone too. This sexy hormone is made in the ovaries, adrenal glands and fatty tissue in women. And unlike oestrogen, testosterone levels in women rise as they approach and after they hit the menopause. In fact, you might be amazed to know women over fifty have as much testosterone as young women and that your testosterone becomes more powerful in your body as you get older.

This is because a substance called sex-hormone-binding globulin (SHBG) binds to, and inactivates, up to 99 per cent of testosterone in a young woman's body. Levels of

SHBG drop by about 50 per cent between your twenties and your late forties, and this allows testosterone to become 'free' or more available for your body to use Also, though your ovaries stop making oestrogen at menopause, they continue to make testosterone. At the same time, the drop in oestrogen adds to the power of testosterone. This means post-menopausal women may actually have more free testosterone than men of the same age. This sex steroid hormone wakes up the libido (well, hello!). But it also causes some physical changes such as the odd hair on the chin, a deeper, huskier voice and changes in the way our fat is distributed. Unfortunately it is associated with driving fat to the waist, hence the change in shape we call 'middle-aged spread'. The rise in free testosterone is also why some women in their late thirties and forties develop a resurgence of spots and oily skin. That dreaded adult acne.

According to research in 2010 for the US Study of Women's Health Across the Nation, this rise in free testosterone causes an increase in visceral fat too. This is the kind of fat that wraps around your internal organs in the torso. Visceral fat increases inflammation in the body and this in turn raises the risk of various diseases. But if too much testosterone is a problem, so is too little. And some women are more at risk of deficiency than others. For example, women who have had their ovaries removed as part of a hysterectomy have half the testosterone of women with intact ovaries.

A study in the British Journal of Dermatology in 2012 found that women with too few 'male hormones' had thinning hair. Giving testosterone therapy led to increased hair growth – where they wanted it! – for 63 per cent of participants. Testosterone lifts mood, and may help reverse reduced muscle size and weaker bones, which are common in post-menopausal women. And in 2013 an exciting new study from Monash University in Australia found that testosterone gel boosted memory and learning in post-menopausal women. Lush hair and a sharper brain? What woman could resist?

DHEA

Made in the adrenal glands, DHEA is known as the 'mother hormone' as it can – ta da! – turn into our other sex hormones, such as oestrogen and testosterone. Production peaks in your mid-twenties, when DHEA is the most abundant hormone in your body.

From your early thirties, your DHEA level steadily declines, so the average seventy-year-old has only 20 per cent of the DHEA of her younger self. Because DHEA converts to key hormones as your body needs them, it is important in creating and maintaining youthfulness and lean muscle mass, in combating stress and protecting the brain, and it can also help you lose weight.

Melatonin

Made in the pineal gland in the brain, melatonin is a sleep and body-clock regulator and a powerful mood booster and antioxidant. Melatonin works with your biological clock by telling your brain when it is time to sleep, though it's worth noting that melatonin does not increase your need for sleep or make you sleep longer.

Melatonin is called the 'vampire hormone' because it is produced primarily in darkness and inhibited by light. Levels of melatonin increase in the middle of the night and gradually fall as the night turns to morning, so exposure to light before bed can push your biological clock in the wrong direction. Due to physical changes, melatonin levels fall, which can cause sleeplessness. (There'll be more on this in the Sleep Chapter on p. 77.)

Melanocyte-Stimulating Hormone

This is a collective name for several hormones produced by the skin, pituitary gland and hypothalamus in response to UV radiation or sunlight. It plays a role in stimulating cells called melanocytes to produce the pigmentation that makes our eyes, hair and skin the colour they are, and which also makes us tan in the sun. This colour protects cells from the DNA damage that can lead to skin cancer, but it has other roles, too. It can suppress our appetite by acting on receptors in the hypothalamus in the brain, which is probably one of the reasons we tend to want to eat less in the summer. It fights inflammation, and affects the release of the hormone aldosterone, which controls salt and water balance in the body and is believed to affect how sexy we feel – and we do feel sexier in the summer, don't we?

In short, hot weather boosts hormones that makes us feel hot! But if you're planning to boost your levels by getting out in the sun, remember, you don't feel or look sexy with sunburn – ouch!

Thyroid Hormones

The thyroid gland at the front of your neck produces the thyroid hormones thyroxine (T4) and, in smaller quantities, triiodthyronine (T3). These hormones are vital to every cell in your body, and control your metabolism, mood, weight, temperature and appearance. In fact, they influence over 300 different targets in your body. An overactive thyroid leads to hyperthyroidism, which causes anxiety, agitation and weight loss, while hypothyroidism, a loss of thyroid hormones, affects at least 10 per cent of women over sixty – and probably many more – causing weight gain, tiredness, mental confusion, depression and the thinning and coarsening of hair and eyebrows. You may feel cold, have puffy skin, muscle pain and weakness that can lead to falls. Pregnancy and childbirth can trigger a period of hyperthyroidism, which then leads to long-term hypothyroidism post-menopause.

If you lost a lot of weight straight after having kids and felt hyper and anxious, followed by a period when you felt exhausted and depressed, you may well have had post-partum hyperthyroidism, a condition that is often misdiagnosed as post-natal depression. If the symptoms sound familiar, and remember, they can be mild or severe and affect up to 25 per cent of women, be particularly vigilant about hypothyroidism and see your GP regularly for blood tests.

Thyroid problems are often misdiagnosed, but a simple at-home temperature test can help you discover if you are low in thyroid hormones:

- Shake down an oral thermometer and place it next to your bed before going to sleep.
- As soon as you wake up, pop the thermometer under your armpit and leave it there for ten minutes while you lie still.
- Record the temperature. If it's below normal rising temperature (36.5–36.8°C) for two consecutive days, you are very likely to be hypothyroid.
- During your menstrual years, your temperature is best measured on the second and third days of your period after flow starts.
- If you think you are hyper- or hypothyroid, you need to see your GP or a specialist doctor as you may require long-term medical treatment.

Cortisol

Cortisol is produced in the adrenal gland and is the hormone that responds to stress. It's known as the 'stress hormone', but it's more accurate to say that it's an 'anti-stress' hormone, as it is the body's defence against stress and inflammation. It is vital to our health, controls blood pressure, is essential for our immune response and gives our body energy when we need it – as in the fight-or-flight response – by releasing sugar into the bloodstream. However, too much cortisol is dangerous.

The only hormones that increase from our mid-thirties

onwards are the 'catabolic' ones, such as cortisol. Catabolic means that they break down muscle tissue, which is bad news for our strength, metabolism and body shape. Excess cortisol is also responsible for fat storage, increasing blood pressure and blood sugar, and reducing immune responses. See the Stress chapter to find ways to reduce excess cortisol, p.55.

Growth Hormone

Human growth hormone (HGH) is made in the pituitary gland and is released in pulses in the early stages of sleep. It helps stimulate your body to grow, and is also believed to be important for tissue repair, muscle growth, healing, brain function, physical and mental health, bone strength, energy and metabolism. From your thirties onwards, your all-important growth hormone naturally decreases by about 14 per cent per decade, until it plateaus in your sixties. This fall results in less skin elasticity, slower recovery time from injuries, brittle bones and less muscle. Other effects include low sex drive, poorer blood sugar control and immune system, and a worsening memory. It may be the primary factor in hormonal ageing.

Pregnenolone

Never heard of it? You are not alone. Yet despite being one of the least-known hormones, pregnenolone can be converted into either DHEA or progesterone and then converted into one or more other hormones, for example, cortisol, testosterone and oestrogens.

19

Made from cholesterol in your body, it seems to help maintain your hormone balance, and it declines with age. You have 60 per cent less pregnenolone at seventy-five than you do at thirty-five.

Pregnenolone produces other hormone-like substances in the body, which can greatly improve our resistance to stress. It works as a 'neuro-hormone', helping to balance moods and emotions and enhancing your memory. It may also be responsible for your youthful skin.

Adiponectin

This is a hormone secreted from your fat cells. It regulates insulin function and reduces inflammation in your circulatory system. High levels are associated with low body fat. If you get fatter, your levels of adiponectin fall, making you more at risk for insulin resistance. Insulin resistance occurs when your body cells lose sensitivity to insulin, the hormone that works to clear sugar from the blood. This makes the body produce more and more insulin, while blood sugar levels remain stubbornly high. Left untreated, this condition leads to weight gain, diabetes and inflammation. Eating more fibre, taking fish oils and exercising can help raise adiponectin levels, while vitamin K activates a protein called osteocalcin, which increases production of adiponectin.

Using the following tables, we reveal the link between your symptoms and hormonal changes, enabling you to become your own hormone doctor.

HOW HORMONES AND MINERALS CAN AFFECT YOUR ENERGY LEVEL

Slow Thyroid	Tired when waking up and when resting. That tiring sensation fades away during morning and when busy and active.
Low Oestrogens	Permanently tired, all day long.
Low Testosterone	Permanently tired, all day long, but increasing when physically active.
Low Cortisol	Extremely tired in the evening, with increased peaks in case of stress.
Low HGH	Intense tiredness in the evening. Difficulty in staying awake after midnight. Feeling it's impossible to recover the morning after.
Low Aldosterone	Tired when standing up.
Low Iron	Mainly tired in the evening, but feeling fatigued all day long.
Low Vitamin B12	Constant fatigue, with peaks during physical and mental activity.
Low Co Q10	Muscular tiredness.
Low Magnesium	Muscular tiredness that increases with stress.

HOW HORMONES CAN AFFECT
YOUR SKIN AND WRINKLES

Lack of HGH and Testosterone (DHEA)	Drooping eyelids.
Low Cortisol and Insulin	Hollow cheeks, lack of fat.
Low HGH	Thin lips, thinner jaws, falling cheeks.
Low Oestrogens	Thighs too soft, fat above knees, thin transparent skin, falling breasts.
Low Oestrogens and Testosterone	Crumpled upper lip.

HOW HORMONES CAN AFFECT
YOUR BODY FAT

Puffed-up face in the morning, swollen cheeks and eyelids	Slow thyroid
Face like a balloon	Too much cortisol, not enough HGH and testosterone
Buffalo's neck	Too much cortisol, not enough HGH, testosterone and T3
Heavy, big breasts	Low progesterone, eventually low HGH and testosterone
Big belly (man and woman)	Low DHEA, eventually low testosterone
Big bottom and thighs	Too much insulin, low cortisol, T3, HGH and testosterone
Cellulite	Low testosterone and HGH
Big calves	Sign of slow thyroid
Bloated legs and ankles	Often slow thyroid, sometimes too much aldosterone

Take Control!

- Falling levels of hormones cause ageing.
- Your hormones work together for optimum health.
- Information is power! Understanding your hormones is the key to staying younger.

'There is no more creative force in the world than the menopausal woman with zest.'
Margaret Mead, anthropologist

2. Take Control: Attitude

When we sat down to write this book, we were excited about sharing the science of staying youthful. We wanted to give you all the latest news on how diet, exercise, stress and sleep affect your crucial hormone balance, and to show you how you could start to reverse your own ageing journey in a way that was fun, not dull, indulgent, not punishing – and just plain enjoyable. But the more we talked about how we felt about getting older and, crucially, the more we talked about the fabulous, amazing, age-defying women who have totally inspired us, the more we realized one thing, and that's this: it's all about the attitude. Yup, as the ageless gals from Bananarama once put it, 'It ain't what you do it, it's the way that you do it.' Because while Botox® can take away your wrinkles, it won't make you seem a day younger if you're a hor-moaner. That's our word for women who are constantly whiny, negative and poor-me-ish. They whinge about their ailments, complain about 'young people today', yet never stop griping about getting older.

Ugh! There is absolutely no point in getting your hormones sorted if you don't have the right attitude. And the results are not just mental but physical. There is nothing, absolutely nothing, more youthful than having a positive outlook and being open to new experiences. Did you know that doing new things literally rewires the brain and keeps it looking – in scans – like a younger brain? A 2012 study of rats at the Max Planck Florida Institute, published in the journal *Neuron*, found that new sensations rewired fibres that supply the input to the cerebral cortex, the part of the brain that's responsible for how we experience sensations, control our bodies, and our thinking and understanding. And this happened in late rat adulthood, not when the brain was young and still forming. (Yes, we know, rats, but oddly enough most people tend to be unwilling to let scientists poke about in their sliced-up brains.) One of the authors of the paper, neuroscientist Marcel Oberlaender Ph.D., said, 'We were able to demonstrate that the brain can rewire, even at an advanced age. This may suggest that if one stops learning and experiencing new things as one ages, a substantial amount of connections within the brain may be lost.'

Another 2006 study published in the journal *Progress in Brain Research* – 'Brain Plasticity and Functional Losses in the Aged: Scientific Bases for a Novel Intervention', Mahncke, H. W., Bronstone, A., Merzenich, M. M. – found that the less our brains do, the more they degrade, and the more we challenge ourselves, the more powerful they become. What does this prove? It's not our age that makes our brains less effective, it's thinking we are too old to learn and do new things.

To be honest, if there's one thing we would love to ban, it's women saying they are 'too old' for anything. What the hell does that even mean? When we came to write this book, Susie and Leah discussed their personal inspirations for ageing in kick-ass style. Leah cited her inspirational mother. Susie, her friend Jackie Curbishley. Looking around, it wasn't hard to find other inspirational women – apart from the political and business Titans we mentioned earlier. Take Gladys Burrill, who finished the Honolulu Marathon in Hawaii in 2010 – aged ninety-two. Luxe label Lanvin's creative director Alber Elbaz picked the phenomenally chic dancer Jacquie Murdock to model in an ad campaign, shot by so-hip-it-hurts Steven Meisel – Jacquie was eighty-two. Are they too old? Do you think Elle Macpherson, fifty-something, is too old to wear a string bikini? Do you think she'd care if you said yes? Perhaps they are exceptional women, but we say that what makes them that way is more than the way they work out, eat or look. They are amazing because of the way they think. They don't think they are too old. They don't act their age or buy into the old, outdated and frankly grim stereotypes about how to look and behave over forty, and this means they do more. And the more you do, the younger you become.

But while doing new things is undeniably important, this doesn't mean that as you get older you should give up the things that have always made you feel fabulous. This isn't just our wishful thinking, either. You know how amazing you feel when you get together with old girlfriends or colleagues, drink cocktails in your old haunt and laugh yourself sick reminiscing, or even just listening to the music you loved in your twenties? There's nothing superficial about that buzz. There is solid science that proves that when you feel it, it can actually reverse the ageing process.

Incredible, eh? And we don't just mean that if you act younger you'll feel younger – though you will – but you will look younger and actually be physically more youthful and even live longer.

As psychology professor Ellen Langer says, 'Everybody knows in some way that our minds affect our physical being, but I don't think people are aware of just how profound the effect actually is.'

Langer is the woman who blew this field wide open in 1980 with an amazing study in which elderly, often sick old men in their late seventies or eighties were invited for what she described as a 'week of reminiscence'. She wanted to know whether, if she could put the mind back twenty years, the body would show any changes.

The men were split into two groups. One was told to live as normal, the other was put into a 1959 time warp, with clothes, furniture, music and TV from their youth, and was asked to act as if it really was 1959. Even though the men were frail, there were no grab rails, no ramps and no concessions to old age. Within days the men seemed younger; they stopped using sticks and started playing football. But more astonishingly, within a week – that's just seven days, remember – tests proved that their speed of movement, memory, arthritis, mental ability and even their eyesight and hearing had all improved.

Langer's verdict at the time? 'My own view of ageing is that one can, not the rare person but the average person, live a very full life, without infirmity, without loss of memory that is debilitating, without many of the things we fear.' Isn't that just fabulous and inspiring? And this is not the only amazing bit of evidence about how our minds affect our youthfulness. What we assume are symptoms of ageing, signs that our bodies are breaking down with age, are often simply the result of us subconsciously buying into what other people think about older people. Yes, you are allowing stereotypes and prejudices to poison and literally age you.

So when you reinforce those stereotypes by what you say, do and believe, you make yourself older. How crazy is that? Yet the minute you start to think younger, you instantly become younger. You may think you only get a great haircut and colour away those pesky grey roots so other people think you look younger, but there is an even more profound effect going on in your own body when you look at yourself in the mirror and truly believe you look younger. And it's an effect that other people can see, too.

In a study, researchers showed people photographs of forty-seven women, aged between twenty-seven and eighty-three, before and after a hair appointment. Those who reported feeling younger with their new style, regardless of whether they'd had their hair dyed, actually appeared younger to the independent raters. And do you know the most amazing thing? The women's hair was cropped out of the photo, which means just thinking your hair makes you look younger will make your face appear more youthful. And do you know what else? Those women who thought they looked younger? Their blood pressure went down, too. How incredible is that? This proves that we all subconsciously scan each other's appearance to estimate age. But we also do it to ourselves! If other people think we look older, they treat us as older and we feel and actually become older. But what is even more extraordinary, if *we* look in the mirror and think we look older, that also ages us mentally and physically. And that's the best argument we've heard for a trip to the salon in a long time. Yes, you are worth it.

In studies, people whose age can't easily be guessed by colleagues because they wear a uniform have better health than those whose clothes give away their age, even if they earn a similar amount and have jobs of similar status. Women who have kids later in life live longer than those who have them earlier, probably at least partly because they live a younger lifestyle, see themselves as 'young mums' at an age when they could be gearing up for grannyhood, and hang out with younger friends (they're probably dressing younger, too).

And finally, marrying a younger man helps you live longer. In marriages with a big age gap, younger wives and husbands die earlier, while older ones live longer, probably because a young partner makes you live a younger lifestyle and surrounds you with younger friends. In other words, cougars do more clubbing and less complaining!

So what does this mean for you? First, make sure your self-talk doesn't reinforce those dreary old-age stereotypes. If you find yourself about say, 'Oh, I'm too old to do X or Y,' or, 'I did that stupid thing because I'm so old,' or, 'Oops, senior moment,' just stop it NOW.

It's probably not even true – though it could become true if you don't shut up. Second, quit hor-moaning. Nothing is more ageing, especially if you are dissing the thoughts, behaviour or tastes of people just because they are younger than you. Never, ever use the phrase, 'in my day'. It's toxic! Stay up to date with technology. Refusing to use the internet or get emails, sneering at Twitter, saying you can't work an iPad or not getting a decent phone all screams 'past-it'.

As for physical complaints, if your back hurts or your feet hurt, or you're tired, don't whine – it's so ageing! – do something about it. Get a massage, have a nap, go for a swim. Hor-moaning is catching – like flu – so avoid spending time with hor-moaners, too. If you have a friend who drags you down by complaining about her age, minor ailments and her regrets, Susie's advice is to be open with her and give her a deadline. Say, 'I love you, but all this whinging is a real downer. For the next week, I'm going to listen to all your woes, but after that, I just don't want to hear them. I want to have fun with you, to be positive and celebrate all the great stuff in our lives. It will make both of us feel better.' She might think you are harsh, and be scared at the prospect of breaking the habit of hor-moaning, but you will be doing yourself, and her, a huge favour. If she can't stop, then maybe take a break from spending time with her.

Third, on a more cheerful note, dress youthfully. Stay on trend. Wear things you love, but watch out that your clothes, make-up or hair don't date you. You don't have to be ridiculous, but things like skinny jeans, Converse or Supergas, T-shirts, shorter skirts, black outfits, leather jackets (ideally tan and well worn-in) and heels aren't just for kids, they are for anyone who looks and feels good in them. Please don't disappear in baggy, beige clothes. If in doubt, think Helen Mirren, former French *Vogue* editor-in-chief Carine Roitfeld, Julianne Moore, Joanna Lumley or Susan Sarandon. Not only are they drop-dead sexy, refusing to wear any kind of 'old lady' uniform, they're unafraid of fashion or of revealing the shape of their bodies; it's a look that just oozes confidence.

Speaking of fashion, a word of advice: we love a bit of vintage – give us a beaded bag and we're happy – but part of the charm of vintage on young women can be the contrast between the older style of the clothes and their obvious vibrant youth. If you look in the mirror and see someone dressed head to toe in slightly shabby, old women's clothes, you may subconsciously take on outdated messages about age and appropriate behaviour, so subtly changing your behaviour and the way people react to you. So wear your (immaculate, flattering) vintage clothes with a modern attitude and flair, and mix with modern items for a look that's fab, not frump.

Finally, we want to pass on Susie's absolutely genius and totally key piece of advice: 'Just stop telling people your age!' No coyly asking people to guess. No girlish hinting. Don't even put your age on job applications or CVs. If people ask your age, don't tell them. This has nothing to do with being ashamed of your age. We agree (sheepishly) that the real reason so many of us do the hints and the big reveal is actually because we look good and dress youthfully and love that über-flattering moment when people gasp and say, 'God, you can't be that old! You look so young!'

But remember, once people know your age, they won't forget it, and if you're over forty, your age will come with a lot of horrible stereotypes that they will probably believe in, even if they don't know they do. They might start to treat you differently, and that will only make you feel older. And as we now know for sure, feeling older makes you old, and feeling and thinking young can actually make you younger.

Which do you choose?

Inspirational Women

About thirty years ago, Susie met an amazing woman who at the time was managing the rock band The Who. She was a tiny little thing, blonde and gorgeous with so much energy, and Susie, even at 6 feet tall, often had to run to keep up with her. She was immersed in the world of rock 'n'roll, and had the most positive attitude towards everything. Fiercely intelligent and political, she became a mentor to Susie, and to a lot of other women as well.

Her name is Jackie Curbishley and she was the first person to make Susie aware of the power of positive thinking, healthy eating and the effect of hormones on your body.

At almost seventy years old, she still has more energy than the average thirty-year-old. She never stops learning and doing new things, and is truly an inspiration. We asked her to contribute a bit of her story and here are a few lines from her:

It is a rare woman, indeed, who doesn't wish to hold back the years. My mother was one such rare woman. She stopped wearing a bra when she was in her fifties and, as far as I know, never used anything but soap and water on her skin. It showed. By the time she was in her mid-sixties she was deeply lined and could tuck her breasts into her waistband. I loved her dearly, but I vowed not to follow her example.

At the age of fourteen, I read about 'beauty routines' in a copy of *Woman's Own* and learned never to sleep in make-up and never to sleep without a night cream. I used a cheap wipe-off cleanser, Nivea was my night cream (it was all I could afford from my pocket money) and I made my own toner from witch hazel diluted with water. I was always told how lucky I was to have such good skin.

I started to investigate hormones and their effect on the ageing body when I passed fifty and found myself in the menopause. After a brief flirtation with hormone replacement therapy, I eventually discovered DHEA (a bio-identical hormone) and melatonin (the substance that regulates sleep, but declines as we age). I've been using them both every night for almost twenty years.

Some years later I discovered HGH (human growth hormone), after reading a glowing testimonial by the film director Oliver Stone. He said it had changed his life, given him back his vitality and worked like a charm. He was taking it in injection form, which wasn't available in the UK, so I researched like mad about the alternatives to taking injections of HGH and discovered that a combination of L-lysine, L-arginine and glutamine could do the trick. I sailed through my menopause using DHEA and the amino acids listed above, and I still, at seventy, take the same combination of hormone supplements every day.

Susie was so impressed with what I was taking and the effects it had had on me that she began her mission to produce and turn her clients on to what I was using, and indeed, took them herself.

These natural supplements remain the bedrock of my regime today. I eat little and often, mainly vegetables and raw food, though I do have the odd indulgence of dessert and wine – I am only human after all.

I dance, sing, paint, write, stretch, practise yoga, run around the globe meeting new people and, at seventy, I feel my life is just beginning. My friends tell me I look pretty good, too. I flirt like mad – I'm still partial to a handsome face – and I wake up each morning, touch my toes ten times, do a simple yoga workout and look for something to laugh about. They tell me that seventy is the new fifty. Well, in my mind seventy is the new thirty!

Jackie Curbishley

'"The water doesn't know how old you are." This can hold true for the basketball court, the golf course, the office and so on. Just because you are a certain age doesn't mean that you can't achieve your goals or dreams.

Capitalize on what you *can* do, not what you *can't* do, and more than likely you'll amaze yourself. With passion comes desire, and with desire comes achievement.'

Darra Torres, twelve times Olympic medallist who, at the age of forty-one, became the oldest swimmer ever to earn a place on the US Olympic team

Take Control!

- Stop telling people your age. 'Old enough' is a perfectly good answer. Take your age off your CV.
- Hang out with younger people. It could help you live longer, and weddings are more fun than funerals.
- Making yourself look younger could be of more benefit to you than to anyone else. Don't think vanity is a bad thing. Book that hair appointment now. Buy those ah-maz-ing shoes.
- Stop whining about your age and ailments and do something positive instead. Encourage your friends to do the same.
- Get a project. Always have things to look forward to and be passionate about, be it a house, a job, a holiday or a man.
- Never think there's anything you can't do because you are 'too old'. Do stuff you love, that makes you feel passionate, happy and alive. A bonus?

A 2011 study in the journal *Psychology and Aging* found that a smile takes two years off your age.
- As the totally fabulous writer Nora Ephron put it, 'Be the heroine, not the victim, of your own life.' In other words, just stop hor-moaning.

'Women may be the one group that grows more radical with age.'
Gloria Steinem

3. Take Control: Body Changes

While we're on our soapboxes, we don't think women get anything like enough information about the vital transitions we make in mid-life. In fact, we are constantly being cornered by women desperate to ask us dozens of questions about their own hormonal change. We think that's wrong. Knowledge is power! The more you know about what's happening to your body, the more you can do to ensure your transition is smooth and easy. Remember, by 2030 it's estimated that women's average life expectancy will be eighty-seven (we're planning to live to a hundred, by the way), so the start of this change comes only halfway through your life and affects every one of us. This is not a minor issue! So let's look at what happens, and how the changes in your hormones affect your mind and body.

Peri-Menopause Explained

The menopause – the time when your periods stop for ever – never really just happens out of the blue, even though for some lucky women it can feel like that. Inevitably, there are years before your periods stop when your hormones are changing, often without your even noticing. In fact, at least at the beginning, you will have regular periods, feel fine and look as young as ever. So how does it start? The peri-menopause may start any time after thirty-five, or even earlier in a few rare cases, though you often won't notice symptoms until you are well into your forties. It's worth mentioning that smoking can cause you to hit the menopause up to three years earlier, and so can thyroid problems (worth remembering if you or someone you know hopes to have a later-life baby). In the last two years before your menopause, hormonal changes tend to become more obvious, and you may get what we think of as menopausal symptoms, such as hot flushes.

This time in your life, from the first hormone shifts until a year after your final period, can last up to ten years and is called the peri-menopause. It can be a worrying, confusing, even frustrating time. Some women feel sad that the fertile period of their life is ending, especially as we associate fertility with youth. Maybe you still half-wish you could have another baby, or are actively trying for one? But you can also feel the same sadness if you've had your children or never wanted kids at all. It's the end of an era, a big transition to make, and most women are pretty much guaranteed to feel wobbly at some point, especially with their hormones going crazy. And it's only made worse if you don't know what's going on, leading you to feel power-less to improve matters.

In fact, the peri-menopause is not an event, but a process, with five distinct stages.

NOTE: If you notice changes in your cycle, such as spotting, heavy periods and change in cycle length, see your GP. It is not unusual for changes to be brought on, or worsened, by medically treatable problems such as thyroid disorders, ovarian cysts or fibroids.

The Stages of the Peri-Menopause Explained!

Remember, everyone's peri-menopause is different. Symptoms will vary, and every stage can last a different time for each woman.

Phase 1

At this point you still have pretty regular periods, but their length may start to change quite subtly. They can become longer, but more usually they become shorter, maybe lasting three days instead of four. Your cycle – the time from the first day of one period to the first day of the next – may shift to become shorter, too, with periods arriving, say, every twenty-five days instead of every twenty-eight, or starting to appear a little later. These changes are caused by changes in two hormones that control ovulation and the menstrual cycle, follicle-stimulating hormone (FSH), which triggers ovulation, and inhibin B, which suppresses FSH. They work as a kind of ovulation tag team. Shifts in levels of these have been shown by studies to be the first symptom of the menopause occurring.

You may also find your breasts become very sore and tender, especially premenstrually. You might find yourself on the internet, looking up an extra supportive exercise bra. You might develop mood swings, finding yourself unexpectedly furious or tearful, experience fluid retention, and either develop PMT for the first time, or find it gets worse. You might gain weight, migraines can happen and some women will have heavier periods. Happy days! On the other hand, you may not look or feel old, your fertility will be falling, but won't have gone, and you might simply put your symptoms down to being busy and tired.

Phase 2

Your cycles are still fairly regular, but you might start to experience heavy bleeding and even flooding. Periods may start to become very painful, with severe cramps. You might miss the odd period. You might find you get migraines for the first time, triggered by hormone fluctuations. Or your migraines might get worse – the good news is that two-thirds of migraine sufferers get fewer and less painful migraines after the menopause. Night sweats might start to appear. These tend to occur in the early hours and are worse in the days before your period – you might just assume you have a virus. You could suffer severe PMT. Your oestrogen levels will be high, if erratic, so breast tenderness and other Phase 1 symptoms will continue and could get worse. Ow!

Phase 3

Your periods are now getting more unpredictable. Sometimes they are short, sometimes long. The gaps between them become more irregular. Sometimes you'll have long gaps, sometimes short ones, and sometimes you'll skip a cycle or two. Your oestrogen levels are intermittently high, normal and even sometimes low. As the levels get more erratic, you might start to get sweats or hot flushes during the day as well as in the night, but these will probably be mild. Night sweats might get worse, but will still tend to appear premenstrually. You may develop gynaecological symptoms, such as urinary tract or yeast infections, and you may also find fibroids, which you might expect to shrink as you get older, but actually grow under the influence of oestrogen surges. At least half your menstrual cycles are 'anovulatory', which means that no egg is produced. As cortisol levels rise, you may experience episodes of foggy thinking. The big M is on its way.

Phase 4

By now your periods are getting very irregular, lighter and much less frequent, though you may also get spotting between periods. You could have as few as four periods a year. You might even miss as many as six periods, think you've gone through the menopause, only to find they start up again when you least want them to. You might have more frequent hot flushes and night sweats, which are no longer tied to your menstrual cycle. You will be ovulating in fewer than half of your cycles. Oestrogen levels are finally falling. Yes, it's true. Oestrogen levels only really start to drop around six months to a year before the menopause proper. Night sweats could mean you buy more sheets and spend more time with your washing machine. On the upside, there are fewer tampons to buy!

Phase 5

This phase begins with your last period and lasts for a year. Of course, you won't know it's your last period as it happens, but you might start to get PMT and cramps with no period; worse, hot flushes and night sweats. Your oestrogen levels are now falling fast. On the bright side, that awful bloating, breast tenderness and moodiness may start to lift. For many women, as the peri-menopause rollercoaster ride draws to a halt, things really start to improve and happiness levels rise. Welcome to the menopause!

Oestrogen Dominance – The Peri-Menopausal Problem

Now, many of you may have noticed something unexpected in what you've just read. Often women in the peri-menopause assume their woes are down to their oestrogen levels plummeting as their ovaries give up the ghost. You may even have read that the peri-menopause is a time when your oestrogen levels slowly and evenly tail off. Well, as you now know, oestrogen levels only fall permanently right at the end of the peri-menopause, so low oestrogen is not a problem. On the contrary. Though levels are fluctuating, on the whole, studies show that women in the peri-menopause tend to have high levels of oestrogen overall, often higher than when they were young, juicy and fertile. So what are you short of? Progesterone! As you now know, changes to the hormones FSH and inhibin B, which trigger the peri-menopause, mean that more of your cycles become 'anovulatory', meaning you don't release an egg that month, so you couldn't conceive if you wanted to. Ovulation is the trigger that causes your body to release progesterone.

During your menstrual cycle, your ovaries produce a surge of oestrogen, which peaks around day twenty-one, and this should be balanced by a peak in progesterone at the same time. So what happens if it doesn't? If oestrogen levels rise without the balance of progesterone, it creates a situation called unopposed oestrogen, or 'oestrogen dominance', a syndrome that might equally be called 'progesterone deficiency'. In fact, during the peri-menopause, progesterone levels decline 120 times more rapidly than oestrogen levels. And with fat-accumulating cortisol also on the rise, it's no surprise that middle-aged spread is a problem even before the menopause kicks in. Oestrogen-dominance symptoms also include foggy thinking, depression and forgetfulness.

What are Hot Flushes and How Can You Treat Them?

No, it's not hot in here. And yes, it is you. Hot flushes are probably the most well-known peri-menopausal symptom. They affect up to 80 per cent of women around the menopause transition, usually starting towards the end of the peri-menopause and lasting one or two years into the menopause proper, though they can last much longer. At night, they wake us up at 3 a.m., our hearts racing, tangled in soggy sheets. By day, they ruin our make-up, make our shirts stick to our backs and send us rushing to open windows and turn off the heating as our younger colleagues shiver (hey, suck it up, it will happen to you, too, one day). Often you'll get a slightly sick feeling of dread that means a flush is on its way, at other times they'll just be a lovely surprise! The intense feeling of searing heat in your upper body usually lasts from thirty seconds to five minutes – the average is four minutes – but what causes them? Yup, it's your hormones.

As oestrogen levels go up and down, this seems to confuse the hypothalamus, the part of the brain responsible for controlling, among other things, your body temperature. We don't know how, but when oestrogen levels drop, this makes the hypothalamus think the body is too hot. Immediately, it sends off a klaxon alert of chemical messengers, particularly epinephrine, with the panicky instruction, 'COOL THIS WOMAN DOWN NOW!' The body obediently responds by getting the heart pumping faster, all the blood vessels in the skin dilate to allow blood to radiate the 'heat' away and your sweat glands spring into action like a sprinkler system. Now you really are hot, though frankly, right now, you feel anything but. Ironic, eh?

Like many other menopausal symptoms, hot flushes are worse in women who have had their ovaries surgically removed, and they are also usually worse in women who smoke.

What Can You Do About Them?

The single most effective treatment for hot flushes is hormone replacement therapy – we'll tell you more about the advantages of that in Chapter 11. However, if you don't want or can't take hormones, alternative medical treatments include selective serotonin reuptake inhibitors (SSRIs), which are a type of antidepressant medicine. These include citalopram, fluoxetine, paroxetine and escitalopram. Some women who took these during the menopause noticed they had fewer hot flushes, a side effect that researchers have confirmed in later trials. Indeed a new drug, Brisdelle, based on paroxetine, has been approved in the US to reduce hot flushes even in women who are not depressed. A serotonin and noradrenaline reuptake inhibitor (SNRI) antidepressant called venlafaxine can also have this effect. Doctors aren't sure how they work, and we know they aren't effective for all women, but if they are, then the result is normally obvious within a week or two, and some doctors will prescribe them for hot flushes. However, side effects include nausea and lack of libido. Gabapentin, a medication used to control seizures and pain, can also help reduce hot flushes, and again a doctor may prescribe this for you. In women for whom they are effective, these medications can cut daily flushes by around 60 per cent. Another possible future form of non-hormonal treatment for hot flushes could be hypnosis. The results of a study, published in *Menopause: The Journal of the North American Menopause Society* in 2012, found that hypnosis can lessen hot flushes by as much as 74 per cent. In addition, two daily servings of soya can reduce the frequency and severity of hot flushes by up to 26 per cent, according to a study published in the same journal in the same year.

For women in the peri-menopause suffering from hot flushes, with or without other peri-menopausal symptoms, Dr Sister recommends the herbal remedies black cohosh and liquorice. Evidence is mixed, but one 2005 study reported by the US government's Office of Dietary Supplements found that women who took 8 mg of black cohosh extract a day in a supplement called Remifemin reported more relief from hot flushes than women taking oestrogen or a placebo pill. The daily rate of hot flushes decreased from 4.9 to 0.7 in the black cohosh group; 5.2 to 3.2 in the oestrogen group; and 5.1 to 3.1 in the placebo group. Scientists aren't quite sure how black cohosh works, but it seems to work like oestrogen in the body, without actually adding oestrogen.

There's a similarly mixed bag of evidence for liquorice, but it's super-safe, and in one study at the University of Southern California, reported at the American Society for Reproductive Medicine's annual conference, women with an average age of fifty-one were given a once-a-day liquorice supplement for a year. There was no improvement for eight months, but then the women found the number of hot flushes fell by 80 per cent, from an average of ten to just two a day. And instead of waking up clammily four times a night, they had just one or two sweating episodes. You can buy liquorice root supplements or use the dried root to make tea. The University of Maryland Medical

Center recommends using 1–5 g of dried liquorice root per cup, up to three times a day.

Caffeine and alcohol tend to make flushes worse, so reducing these and giving up smoking can only help your hot flushes, as well as your general health.

Four Good Reasons to Give Up Smoking Now

Yes, yes, you've heard it before. But if you haven't given up smoking yet, mid-life is the perfect time to stub out the habit. It really is never too late to stop and reap the benefits.

1. Not smoking halves your risk of hot flushes, according to the University of Pennsylvania Perelman School of Medicine.

2. Smoking makes for thinner, weaker bones. According to the US National Institutes of Health, the longer and more you smoke, the greater your risk of fracture in old age. Plus smokers take longer to heal, and that includes their bones.

3. Oestrogen can protect your heart, but after the menopause that protection begins to decrease and, combined with smoking, this pushes the risk of heart disease right up. A study from Harvard Medical School, Boston, published in the *New England Journal of Medicine*, found that women who smoked as few as one to four cigarettes a day had double the risk of suffering a heart attack as those who didn't smoke. The good news? Giving up cuts your risk almost instantly.

4. Collagen is an important part of what keeps skin bouncy, plump and wrinkle-free. Seventy per cent of your skin is collagen. Smoking breaks down collagen, and lack of oestrogen after the menopause can also lead to collagen loss. Smoking just speeds up this process.

The Menopause Explained

Women reach the menopause, on average, at fifty-two, though the exact age can vary wildly. A menopause before age forty-five is considered early, and a very few women don't get there until they hit their sixties. When it does happen, though, hormone levels change a lot. When your periods finally stop, levels of the sexy little hormone oestrogen, the one that keeps us juicy, lush-haired and plump-skinned, as well as causing all those problems, drop. But just because your periods have ended, it doesn't mean your symptoms have. Hot flushes and mood swings can keep on happening and can even get worse. And it's not just oestrogen levels that fall. Levels of all our hormones drop as we age. And these hormones, which include sex hormones such as oestrogen, progesterone and testosterone, plus our essential growth hormones, control every function of our bodies. For example, oestrogen protects those telomeres we were telling you about earlier. Our hormones also affect our appetite and where we store fat. You know those stubborn pounds we talked about at the beginning? Guess what? They're not all your fault.

In addition, scientists recently found that lower levels of oestrogen affect specific areas of the brain that control body temperature, hunger and thirst. When female rats had their oestrogen levels lowered, their metabolic rates and energy levels plummeted. Not only that, but they turned into fat rats, with the weight going straight to their middles. Sound familiar? Scientists believe that low oestrogen also affects our appetite.

Scientists have found that certain enzymes and proteins that control fat storage in the thighs and abdomen change at the menopause. As oestrogen levels fall, women burn less fat, and their fat cells store more fat, particularly around the middle. Low levels of oestrogen turn on a nasty fat-making enzyme. Known as ALDH1A1, this sneaky enzyme causes us to store fat, particularly the most dangerous type of fat around the internal organs, known as visceral fat, which is linked with type 2 diabetes, heart disease and cancer.

Researchers at the University of Ohio found that normal levels of oestrogen suppressed the effects of the enzyme, but once oestrogen levels fell after the menopause, it was free to wreak havoc, causing weight gain and dumping fat around the middle. So what can you do? The study found that a diet high in unhealthy fats seems to make ALDH1A1 more active, particularly in women, so cutting back on unhealthy fats, such as those in cakes, biscuits and junk food, makes sense. And so does supplementing your hormones, but more about this later.

Another reason you may change shape at this point in your life is that you tend to lose muscle cells as you age.

And because muscle, unlike fat, burns calories even when we are doing nothing, that's not good news. So where does the muscle go? When you are young and muscle cells get damaged, you can repair them superfast. As you get older that doesn't seem to happen so quickly. This might be because stem cells in the muscles can't respond to damage in the way they did when you were younger, and if damaged muscle cells aren't repaired, they sort of whittle away and die. Decreases in growth hormone, testosterone and oestrogen levels may also account for loss of muscle. All this means you might experience a 4–5 per cent decrease in metabolic rate per decade, and in the first five years after the menopause you can lose 30 per cent of your collagen and up to 20 per cent of your bones.

Post-menopausal women are also more vulnerable to osteoporosis and heart disease. Yes, we know this sounds bad, but remember, there are ways to change your hormone destiny. We are going to show you clever ways to preserve your bones and collagen. And we have some fantastic news – no, really, this honestly is uplifting stuff – many studies have found women's lives change for the better once they are past the menopause. The 2002 Jubilee Report, which looked at the lifestyles of women over fifty, found that 65 per cent reported that they were happier. Why? Well, 76 per cent of post-menopausal women said their health was better, 75 per cent said they had more fun, and 93 per cent said they had more independence and more choice in everything from work to leisure pursuits.

Many women worry that they will feel less sexual once their baby-making years are over, but for many women, freed from the hormonal havoc of the peri-menopause, the reverse happens. And hormone supplements can help. Half of women on HRT report improvements in their sex lives following the menopause, compared with 18 per cent of those not taking hormones. And remember, you don't necessarily have to suffer all these peri-menopausal symptoms. The key to avoiding them is to adopt the healthy-living ideas we suggest in this book, together with a positive attitude, which studies show makes a massive difference. You are a gorgeous grown-up with confidence, intelligence and fabulous life experiences. Enjoying good food, exercise, stress reduction, sleep, friends and lots of lovely fun can mean your forties and fifties mark the start of the best years of your life.

Take Control!

- Eat more cruciferous vegetables, such as broccoli, cauliflower, kale, spinach, sprouts and cabbage. They contain a nutrient called indole-3-carbinol, which has been shown to help reduce the body's load of excess oestrogens. Try to eat two to three servings a day.
- Eat citrus fruits. They contain D-limonene, another substance shown to help with oestrogen 'detoxification'. Eat one serving a day.
- Boost your intake of soluble fibre. This type of fibre is mainly found in fruit and vegetables, and binds to excess oestrogen in the digestive system,

carrying it out of the body. Apples, pears, citrus fruits, strawberries and oats are rich sources.

- Cut your intake of caffeine. Studies show that two or more cups of coffee a day can increase oestrogen levels.
- Drink less alcohol, as this increases oestrogen levels.
- Keep your weight at a healthy level. Remember, fat cells make oestrogen, which right now will just add to your oestrogen overload.
- To rebalance oestrogen dominance, natural progesterone supplements can dramatically improve the peri-menopausal symptoms – we'll talk more about them later.
- The peri-menopause is a journey, not an event.
- Oestrogen levels tend to go up, not down, but progesterone falls for ten years before the menopause.
- Oestrogen only falls permanently at the menopause.
- Not every woman will struggle at this time.
- For most women, the menopause is a fabulous new beginning – and that includes for their sex lives.

'The hardest years in life are those between ten and seventy.'
Helen Hayes, seventy-three

4. Take Control: Stress

How Getting Calm Can Reverse Ageing, Make You Lose Weight and Make You Smarter

Admit it, it's easy to feel proud of your stress levels. Sounds crazy? Can you honestly say you've never felt a glimmer of pride when you've told someone how 'busy' or even how 'stressed out' you are? After all, this proves how important and in demand you are, and how hectic and interesting your life must be.

A crazy schedule shows you're still young, hot and in demand, right? Wrong. Stress is toxic. Stress makes you old, fat, tired and slow-witted. It kills your libido, stops you sleeping, makes you irritable and hard to be around and increases your blood pressure. Not only that, it's linked to just about every serious illness, from heart disease to cancer.

Why? It starts with hormones. Stress causes a cascade of chemical reactions. One of them is the release of cortisol, which fuels the blood with energy in the form of sugar, enabling us to flee from potential dangers. This was fine when we needed that sugar rush to, say, run away from predators, as the minute we escaped from the sabre-toothed tigers our cortisol would drop and we'd be OK. These days there are fewer sabre-toothed tigers, and more tax bills, bad dates, rows with husbands, deadlines and overdrafts.

Worrying about stuff like this means your cortisol levels stay chronically high. Stress feels good at first because your body's first reaction to stress is to pump out the hormone adrenaline, which gives a rush of energy and a mental high. You don't feel hungry, you don't feel tired, you don't feel pain. You feel strong and brave. Enough adrenaline can make you feel practically superhuman.

But – and it's a big but – as the adrenaline fades, cortisol steps in, and cortisol takes a lot longer to fade away. If it's triggered by constant mini-bursts of adrenaline, it will stick around for even longer and in higher concentrations, and too much cortisol makes you feel anxious, worried and negative. It also stops your brain from laying down a new memory, or from recovering your existing memories, by damaging your hippocampus, a part of the brain that's vital to memory.

To your body, this hormone cascade signals an emergency, so naturally it puts other functions on hold to conserve energy. You know, pointless stuff like growth, reproduction and your immune system. You don't want sex. You get ill. And you look, well, frankly terrible.

As cortisol levels rise, the blood flow to your skin is cut back. Result? You look pale and grey. Cortisol also increases oil in your skin, causing breakouts; and it messes with the skin's natural barrier, a coating of good bacteria that keeps infection at bay. Without it, we are more prone to spots, redness, even eczema and psoriasis.

The Stress/Fat Connection

To get rid of the cortisol-induced sugar in our blood, our body produces a ton of the hormone insulin, which mops it up. But insulin has another effect on our body. It's known as 'the fattening hormone' because it's proven to increase our appetite and encourage our body to store fat.

Also, stress makes many of us indulge in comfort eating, and studies show it primes the brain to want high-fat, high-calorie food. It actually shrinks the prefrontal cortex, the part of the brain associated with problem-solving, coping with change, emotional processing and regulation, impulse control (aka grabbing an apple instead of a doughnut) and regulating your glucose and insulin levels.

Plus, remember how we talked about the way your shape might change in mid-life? About how these hormone changes might mean you find yourself gaining weight around the waist? Well, stress can do this, too.

Scientists have found that too much cortisol can mess with fat storage and lead to a spike in visceral, or internal, belly fat in stressed-out women. That's right, chronic stress contributes to making you fat around the middle. And this stress belly fat doesn't just sit there getting in the way when you are trying to do up your jeans, it's alive!

Abdominal fat cells appear to be particularly active, pouring out hormones and chemicals, including chemicals that promote insulin resistance, a condition that causes the body to have high blood sugar and retain fat, which in turn can lead to diabetes. Visceral fat also releases substances called cytokines, which cause inflammation throughout the body – we'll talk more about this later – inflammation that is seriously bad news, making you fat, old and ill. Basically, it's not something you want to encourage.

The Stress/Age Connection

Let's return to telomeres, those protective caps on the ends of our thread-like chromosomes that play such a vital part in ageing. When our telomeres get too short, our cells stop working, then die. And guess what makes our telomeres shorten? You've got it. S – T – R – E – S – S.

Researchers looked at women in mid-life and older with a common form of anxiety, and found that the women had significantly shorter telomeres. In fact, they had telomeres that were similar to those seen in women six years older. Stress had prematurely aged them, at the deepest cellular level, by six entire years.

How? An enzyme called telomerase protects our telomeres, and stress may reduce our levels of telomerase. High blood sugar also causes glycation, which means that cells become stiff and damaged. Skin cells are particularly vulnerable to glycation, and this leads to skin ageing. Diabetics, who have badly controlled blood sugar, tend to look older than their years, with more wrinkles and duller, yellower skin. High cortisol even causes our skin to produce less hyaluronic acid, the skin's natural moisturizer.

All this should convince you that stress is truly toxic. We may even have stressed you out a bit by talking about it, in which case, um, sorry. But the good news is, you can beat stress and get your hormones back in balance. Amazingly, you may even make those poor stress-shortened telomeres grow longer.

Watch out for these warning signs that your stress levels are getting out of control

Your body's stress signals:

These are common when you are stressed, but see your GP if you suffer from these to rule out a physical cause.

You start getting headaches and pain behind the eyes, as if someone's tightening an iron band around your head.

You have attacks of shallow breathing, as if you can't quite catch your breath.

You're constantly tired and feel 'drained'.

You have trouble sleeping – either in dropping off, or staying asleep, or both.

Your heart is racing, and it's not because you've found the perfect shoes, or spotted George Clooney.

You're too stressed for sex. Libido, what libido?

You are constantly ill. You get every bug going.

Your skin breaks out, which really isn't fair now you also have wrinkles.

Your back hurts. And so do your shoulders, your knees…

You are grinding your teeth at night, and practically wake up with lockjaw.

You have stomach problems, such as indigestion, feeling sick and your, ahem, bowel habits have changed.

Your emotional stress signals:

Any of these are worrying. Got the lot? You need help fast.

You cry – and not just at sad movies.

You are snappy as a crocodile with toothache. Your partner flinches when you speak. You can't remember when you last had a really good laugh.

You worry constantly, about pretty much everything.

You assume the worst about every situation.

You can't be bothered to see people any more, even your friends.

You feel overwhelmed about everything and find it hard to start, or finish, projects or tasks. You feel panicky.

Your lifestyle stress signals:

You might not recognize these in yourself, but ask your partner or a friend if they apply.

Your house is a mess. You can't face tidying up, let alone making your home beautiful.

You've stopped taking care of your appearance and your health. Who needs lipstick and salad anyway? You've got a stash of unopened letters from the bank, and you have missed payments on your credit card, even if you can afford them.

Your weekend bottle of wine or after-work cocktail is escalating into daily drinking. You need it, yeah? You are smoking more.

You've stopped running, and can't remember when you last made it to your Pilates class.

De-Stress Your Lifestyle

First, take a look at the things you are worried about and get seriously proactive about the things you can change. For example, if you're anxious about money, take a good hard look at your finances. Get out your bank statements, keep a diary of your spending, draw up a spreadsheet and start thinking about where you are wasting money, how you can save and how you can earn more. If you hate your job, do your best to change it.

Even making the decision to take a nagging worry and bringing it into the light can make the problem shrink. Don't get sucked into endless rumination and negative self-talk, such as: 'It's a disaster,' 'I can't go on,' or 'I'll never sort this out.' Why? You can talk yourself into a state of stress, or out of it, just as you choose.

That's not just new-age speak, by the way. A 2005 study of Norwegian school kids found their cortisol levels plummeted if they simply said, 'I can solve this task,' before taking a test. Whereas if they said, 'I'm worried and will have problems solving other tasks, too,' their stress levels went up.

For many of us, stress and worrying are just a bad habit, but if your stress is about stuff you can't change – I mean really can't change, like having a sick child or parent – it's easy to imagine that there is nothing you can do. But a mind–body approach to de-stressing your lifestyle can, and does, work, even for people who have serious problems in their lives. Here's how:

- Try making a self-affirmation. Not quite the same as positive self-talk, affirmations are all about remembering your values. First, make a list of the things that are important to you. Maybe your family, your work, or the 5K you're training for. Then pick one and write about why it matters. Start with 'My family/work/training is important because . . .' This simple task tends to make you feel more positive about yourself and your life, and a 2013 study at Carnegie Mellon University in the US found it boosted creativity and problem-solving as well as reducing stress. Do it as a one-off, or keep a notebook by your bed and make it a regular part of your life.
- Sleep is a vital stress buster. The average fifty-year-old has overnight cortisol levels that are twelve times higher than those of the average thirty-year-old. If you are sleep-deprived you clear cortisol from your system up to six times slower than when you are well rested. It then becomes a vicious cycle, as too much cortisol also makes it harder to sleep well. So you need to try stress-reduction approaches if you suffer from insomnia. Aim for at least seven hours, and forget what they say about early to bed, early to rise. Waking before 7 a.m. seems to be associated with higher cortisol levels.

- So many of us now work a seven-day week. With home internet, 24-hour emails and mobile phones, many of us never truly switch off, as we answer work calls and emails every day of the week. Studies show that taking a day off work reduces stress, so for your mental health and stress reduction, try to take one full day off a week. That means on a Sunday, say, don't read or reply to work emails. Ideally leave your phone at home (we know, we struggle with that too). Taking the odd three-day weekend can have a truly dramatic effect on your stress levels as well.

- Get a massage. Sounds like a cliché? Nope, this has real science behind it. In a 2006 Australian study, high-stress nurses who had a fifteen-minute back massage once a week had lower cortisol levels, lower blood pressure and lower anxiety levels than those who didn't. A 2009 study at the University of Miami School of Medicine showed that a single massage could lower cortisol by an amazing 31 per cent, and raise levels of the happy hormone serotonin by 28 per cent. It also boosts the 'reward chemical' dopamine, which falls post menopause.

- Exercise is super important, too. It boosts levels of endorphins, the feel-good hormone, and also increases levels of the enzyme telomerase. Get some exercise every day, even if it's just walking. A tip: walking outdoors in green surroundings seems to bust stress much more effectively than walking in the grey, polluted city. So if you live in a town, head to the park whenever you can.

- Yoga is fantastic for reducing stress. It has been proven to reduce anxiety, lower blood pressure, improve body image and even cut binge eating as it works on a physical, mental and genetic level. Book a weekly class.

- Have regular hot baths. Warmth seems to help reduce stress, depression and anxiety and increase serotonin levels, and it's also time for you, which we bet you don't get enough of. Add a book and delicious bath oils; try lighting some scented candles, relax and breathe.

- Reading is one of the fastest and easiest ways to reduce stress. In a 2009 study at the University of Sussex, volunteers first had their stress levels and heart rate increased with tests and exercises. Then they tried different ways to reduce stress. Listening to music reduced stress by 61 per cent, going for a walk by 42 per cent, and a cup of tea by 54 per cent, but reading worked best, reducing stress levels by an amazing 68 per cent. Just six minutes of silent reading slowed down the heart rate and reduced muscle tension, and in the end the volunteers had lower stress levels than when they started.

- See your friends. Having a good social network improves longevity more than even having a healthy diet or exercising. Yup, it's that important! A 2010 report by researchers at Brigham Young University and the University of North Carolina in the US collated information from 148 studies, involving more than 300,000 people. They found that the most solitary died on average 7.5 years earlier than the more sociable people, even if they didn't feel lonely. That's almost the difference between smokers and non-smokers.

- Laugh more. See friends who make you laugh, watch a funny movie. Laughter is proven to reduce the stress hormones cortisol by 39 per cent, and epinephrine by 70 per cent, while dramatically increasing levels of lovely, happy serotonin. Laughter also boosts blood flow – with all that gorgeous oxygen and nutrients – boosts your immune system and is fantastically anti-ageing; it's like an internal workout.

Stress-Proof Your Diet

A healthy diet, particularly one high in omega-3 fatty acids, which are found in oily fish such as salmon and mackerel, and omega-6 fatty acids found in nuts and vegetable oils, seems to boost telomerase. It also makes our telomeres grow longer, and helps us become more resistant to stress. (Omega-3s also help reverse a stress belly, if you need more encouragement to eat more of them.)

Fresh vegetables and fruit are essential, while B vitamins are important for helping your body cope with stress, and vitamin D – also present in those all-important oily fish – boosts telomerase. Reduce the amount of caffeine you drink and cut back on alcohol. But you definitely don't have to give up everything you enjoy. Remember, depriving yourself is stressful, and we want your life to be *more* fun, not less. Everything in moderation (most of the time).

Meditate Your Stress Away

A huge part of beating stress is calming the mind. One of the most difficult tasks is sitting still – no telly, no iPhone, no trashy magazines – just you and your thoughts. Ah ha . . . it's those thoughts that keep racing right? Well, the key to finding beauty within is to take time out of your day to observe your mind, shut off your thoughts, take in conscious breaths and be still – otherwise known as meditation.

Meditation – sounds all a bit daunting? I know what

you're thinking: it's not for me. I don't have enough time. I've got kids – no can do. Impossible! Stop right there. Meditation can be simple, as long as you understand it and you learn about what works for you.

Researchers say that meditation helps you lower blood pressure, and some medical theorists even claim that it makes you 49 per cent less likely to die from cancer and 30 per cent less likely to die from cardiovascular disease. Studies show it actually lengthens those telomeres. Plus, there's the added bonus of alleviating chronic pain, boosting your immune system and increasing your brain function – sounds better than falling in love. Well, maybe not!

And you don't have to give up hours of your day either. A 2012 study by the University of California in Los Angeles found that as little as twelve minutes of meditation a day over eight weeks can reduce stress and decrease inflammation in the body. Not only that, it changed the response of a staggering sixty-eight genes in the body. How incredible is that? You can download meditation apps to your phone for a quick fix. Just plug in your earphones and meditate anywhere – even on the train (though sadly not while driving!).

Susie has practised transcendental meditation for many years. It's based on the simple premise of keeping your eyes closed in silence, while repeating a word (or mantra) over and over in your mind. Ideally you'd do this for about twenty minutes each day, but even five minutes a day will help your mind and body.

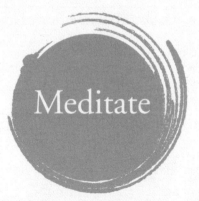

Do-It-Yourself Meditation Using a Mantra

1. Choose a one-syllable word that you like, anything like love, peace, breath, good, etc.

   Find a comfortable chair, prop up pillows on your bed – anywhere where your head is supported and you can sit comfortably. I even meditate on planes.

2. Turn the lights down and try to make sure it's as quiet as possible. (Turn your phone off, so as not to be disturbed.)

3. Breathing slowly in and out with your eyes closed, just keep repeating your word slowly to yourself in your head, trying to follow the rhythm of your breath.

4. As thoughts come into your head, try to bat them away and go back to your word. (Not easy at first but it becomes easier.)

5. Do this for at least twenty minutes a day, if possible, and on an empty stomach.

6. I find first thing in the morning or before dinner at night is perfect.

And Breathe . . .

Breathing is the essence of life. Most of us tend to breathe shallowly, breathing into our chests when we should really be breathing slowly deep into our stomachs. Proper deep breathing will give your body the essential oxygen it needs to function properly, as well as helping to eliminate toxins, particularly carbon dioxide. A study of heart patients found that the optimum healthy breath rate is six breaths a minute. The average resting rate is around fourteen times a minute, so slow down. Here's how:

Whenever you feel stressed, anxious or tired, stop and take the time to inhale and exhale deeply. Relax your shoulders and put your hands on either side of your rib-cage, just below bra-strap level. Spread your fingers wide and take a slow deep breath through your nose (try to count to six), filling up your stomach, ribcage and chest slowly with air – you should feel your stomach and ribcage expanding – then slowly open your mouth and gently let all the air out until there's nothing left. If you can, on the out-breath, pull your navel back towards your spine and squeeze your pelvic floor (more about that later), adding in a bit of stomach work. If you get dizzy, it's because you are not used to taking in that much air. Sit down and repeat. If you do this regularly it will eventually become a habit.

Try the following simple, easy breathing technique, which really works and takes no time at all.

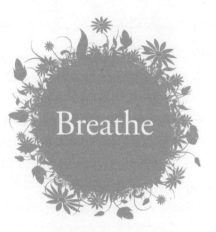

Breathe

Easy Breathing Technique
to Help Reduce Stress

 Sitting straight on a chair, uncross your legs and place your feet firmly on the ground; put your hands on your stomach.

 Breathe in slowly through your nose for the count of six, looking straight ahead. Feel your stomach expand as you breathe in.

 Hold that breath for the count of six, stomach still expanded.

 Then slowly breathe out for the count of six through your mouth, making sure you make an extra effort to really empty your lungs.

 Repeat five times.

Then, put your hands on your rib cage, directly under your bra strap and breathe in slowly for the count of six, expanding your diaphragm.

Hold for the count of six.

Now slowly breathe out to the count of six, making sure you really empty your lungs.

Repeat five times.

Still sitting straight, put your hands on the back of your head, linking your pinkies together. Your elbows will be up in the air.

Breathe in slowly for the count of six as you lower your head (pinkies still touching).

Hold your breath for the count of six while your head is down.

Now slowly, for the count of six, breathe out, fully emptying your lungs as you bring your elbows and head to the start position.

Repeat five times.

Get Mindful

Another way of managing stress is by mindfulness meditation. This technique is all about learning to live in the present and can be done as you go about your everyday life. Instead of racing through a meal, you really savour the look, smell and taste of it. As you walk, you feel the ground beneath your feet, the sensations in your muscles and the feeling of the wind and sun on your body. This is profoundly grounding and can draw you out of the panicky whirl of anxiety so many of us exist in. What's more, a growing body of scientific evidence proves it has a powerful effect on stress, depression and anxiety, and can even reduce chronic pain. One fantastic way to use mindfulness to stop stress in its tracks is to do a 'body scan':

- Start by lying down – it's really easy to do this last thing at night and it only takes a few minutes. All you need to do is focus your attention on each part of your body, as if you were scanning yourself in an MRI machine.
- First, focus on the pressure of your head on the pillow, the sensation of your eyelids on your eyes, the way your heart beats, the heaviness of your legs, right down to the tiniest feelings in your toes.
- Don't judge or worry about the physical feelings, just notice them as interesting sensations. Don't feel you have to do anything. This isn't a relaxation exercise, it's simply about noticing your body and its sensations.
- As you get better at doing this, you can learn to switch on this intense physical focus at will, so you can notice stress-related tension in your forehead, churning in your stomach and jitteriness in your limbs the minute you start to feel stressed. This is often enough to stop the physical sensations in their tracks, and prevent them affecting you emotionally.

Finally, remember the chapter of this book, where we talked about attitude? Stop thinking of yourself as a victim. Stop hor-moaning. Surround yourself with positive people who bring energy and joy to your life. Spending time with others is a fantastic way to prevent stress, but they have to be the right people. In short, if you want a proven way to feel amazing, to lose your mid-life stress belly and actually reverse ageing at the deepest genetic levels, start de-stressing today.

Sarah's Story

As I approached an, ahem, significant milestone birthday, I started to notice some changes in my body. I felt achy and stiff. I skipped a period without being pregnant for the first time ever, yet still got PMT.

My periods were sometimes heavy, sometimes light. There were times I found it hard to focus. At night I'd sometimes feel sweaty and sleep badly. I felt I looked older. But most of all I just felt completely and utterly exhausted. Admittedly, I'd had a difficult year. I'm a lawyer, and an exciting but overwhelming work project had led to my working very long hours, sometimes into the night and at weekends.

Plus I'd had to have a knee operation earlier in the year and I'd been in pain and unable to exercise for nearly a year. I also have three children aged between ten and sixteen. I'd read in a newspaper that every woman of around fifty simply must be suffering from menopausal symptoms, so searching for an answer to my problems I went to see Dr Sister, who had been recommended to me. It was surprising to find a doctor who would just listen to me – my GP wasn't interested at all.

He sent me for a full blood work-up at a London clinic. I was worried about when I should go as my periods had been a bit erratic. He said it didn't matter when in my cycle I went as the results would tell him all he needed to know. At the clinic near Harley Street the nurse was lovely. She took three vials of blood and it was all done in minutes. Amazingly, the full results arrived at Dr Sister's clinic the next day.

I braced myself for the results, thinking I was going to hear that I was pretty much menopausal, though ironically my period arrived on the day of my appointment. I was amazed. Dr Sister explained that not only was I not menopausal, I wasn't even peri-menopausal! All my hormone results were normal. I felt suddenly very youthful, though immediately I vowed to stop being careless with contraception! Dr Sister pointed out that my progesterone was a little on the low side, but still in the normal range. This might be an age-related decline but shouldn't be a problem. I joked that this made me not peri-menopausal, but peri-peri menopausal – like the sauce! I also had slightly high cholesterol, but he told me not to worry and to definitely not consider taking statins. So with hormones ruled out, what was causing my symptoms?

Dr Sister said that in his opinion my problems, including the cholesterol levels, were due to very high stress levels. You might think this means that the tests were pointless, but to me they definitely weren't. I was convinced my problems were due to age, but now that I know that's not the case, I feel extra-motivated to sort out my lifestyle. Dr Sister's prescription is for a proper holiday, some swimming, yoga and to turn off my BlackBerry more often. And that's medicine I'm happy to take.

Take Control!

- Exercise most days. Ideally try yoga, Pilates or walking or running outdoors.
- Eat well. Eat more green vegetables and oily fish. Cut out processed foods.
- Take up meditation of some kind – prayer counts, too – and consider downloading an app to your phone to help you as you learn.
- Sleep more and better.
- Change what you realistically can; learn to cope with what you can't.
- Spend more time with good, positive, friends. Fun is fabulously de-stressing.
- Adopt a positive attitude. It's almost impossible to smile and worry at the same time. Seriously. Go on, try.

'Ageing is not lost youth but a new stage of opportunity and strength.'
Betty Friedan

5. Take Control: Sleep

How Good Are You in Bed?

When it comes to your most important night-time activity – yes, that's sleeping – lots of us rate really badly. We go to bed late, we read our iPads into the small hours, sleep restlessly and wake up tired. Plus for us women, there are particular problems with sleep in mid-life. GPs report that insomnia is the single biggest complaint of menopausal patients. A study has revealed that menopausal women have 61 per cent of their nights disrupted by night sweats.

But that's nothing a caffeine shot won't fix? Wrong. When we skimp on sleep, it's a catastrophe for our hormones. We all know good sleep makes us feel great and look better – it's not called beauty sleep for nothing; be gone those bags! – but sleep is much, much more than a self-indulgent mood booster and beautifier. Sleep is the magic button that switches off the stress hormone cortisol, turns down the heat on your hunger hormones, boosts your metabolism, fires up your brain and reverses ageing. In short, if you don't sleep well, you screw up your hormones and get fat, old, tired and stupid.

No wonder we all feel like hor-moaning.

Sleep Yourself Younger

Scientists now realize that many of the things that look like ageing are in fact the result of chronic sleep deprivation. In a 2004 study at the University of Chicago Medical Center, when young (yup, young, fit and energetic) adults were made to sleep four hours a night instead of eight for just one week, their hormones went haywire. They took 40 per cent longer to normalize their blood sugar levels after a high-carb meal, and their ability to make and respond to the sugar-clearing hormone insulin fell by 30 per cent. They produced less thyroid hormone and more of the stress hormone cortisol; their memories didn't work properly and they couldn't learn or concentrate. Basically their bodies acted as if they were in the early stages of diabetes – or just really, really old.

If lack of sleep can do this to 'bright young things', just imagine what it's doing to you. Eve Van Cauter, Ph.D., professor of medicine at the University of Chicago, told *Time* magazine, 'We suspect that chronic sleep loss may not only hasten the onset but could also increase the severity of age-related ailments such as diabetes, hypertension, obesity and memory loss.'

And, horribly unfairly, it's worse for us women than for men. A 2008 study found lack of sleep is harder on women than men, putting us more at risk of heart disease and diabetes. The study at Duke University in the US found women who didn't sleep well had higher inflammation, cholesterol, insulin and blood sugar levels. In the study, women who found it hard to fall asleep, and took more than half an hour to do so, had the worst risk profile of all.

Chronic excess cortisol also suppresses our immune system, which means it's linked to a host of diseases, including cancer, as well as premature ageing. And as with everything, it's not just quantity that counts but quality. Studies show that even if you rack up the hours in the sack, if the sleep isn't good quality, you won't get the benefits. Cortisol and stress levels soar if you don't sleep well, and in turn, they interrupt your deep sleep, causing multiple 'micro-arousals', which are a lot less fun than they sound, waking you up in the night just enough to interfere with your rest and repair, but not so much that you notice.

Lack of sleep doesn't just make us physically unhealthy. It makes it harder for us to control our impulses, act positively, feel good about ourselves and even empathize with other people. An unsurprising 2013 study from the University of California in Berkeley has shown that couples 'experience more frequent and severe conflicts after sleepless nights'. Without enough sleep, people felt less loving and misjudged each other's emotions, expressions and intentions.

Are You Getting Enough?

Pretty much all of us sleep less than we are designed to. In 1910, the average night's sleep was nine hours. Now it's seven, and falling.

But sleeplessness as you age isn't just the result of bad habits; it's hormonal. Before the menopause, oestrogen works to keep the level of the brain chemical serotonin nice and high. Serotonin isn't just associated with happiness – depressed people have low levels – it naturally reduces levels of the 'wake-up' neurotransmitter acetylcholine in the brain. But when oestrogen levels fall, so do levels of acetylcholine. Women wake up more often in the night and get less deep sleep. Restoring oestrogen using methods such as HRT and supplements can improve sleep and mood in women suffering from hormone-related insomnia.

Also, with age, you produce less of the vital sleep hormone and antioxidant melatonin, which is secreted by the pineal gland in your brain. There are also changes in your brain cells, which are known to regulate your internal clock. Together, this means you miss out on around an extra half hour's sleep a night every ten years. But there's more. As we get older, the amount of time we spend in lovely slow-wave sleep, the deepest, most refreshing part of our sleep cycle, starts to decline.

A healthy young adult spends about a quarter of the night in deep, slow-wave sleep. By the time you reach your forties, you are getting 80 per cent less of this sleep than you did as a teenager. And by the time you hit sixty, you have almost no uninterrupted deep sleep, just short bursts. Scientists aren't sure why this happens, but think it might be connected to a gradual shrinkage of a part of the brain called the middle-frontal lobe as we age. Don't worry, there are solutions, which we will continue to tell you about, exercise being just one of these.

The more deterioration there is, the less slow-wave sleep you experience. So why does that really matter? It's important because slow-wave sleep is when we make and consolidate memories, and this may be connected with memory loss as we age. The less deep sleep we have, the worse we perform in memory tests the next day. This is because in deep sleep, the brain moves memories from the short-term storage of the hippocampus to the long-term storage of the prefrontal cortex at the front of the brain, behind the forehead.

But something else is happening too. During the day our brains take in a lot of information, so brain cells are constantly firing and creating new connections between different parts of the brain. Unfortunately, many of these new connections are irrelevant stuff we don't really need – imagine a cluttered wardrobe full of clothes you never wear – and this 'clutter' of networks makes it harder for us to access the stuff we do need.

Scientists now know that as we sleep our brains are busy sorting through this mess and getting rid of the connections we don't need. Just as sorting out a wardrobe makes it easier and faster to find a useful outfit, this brain de-cluttering strengthens the most vital connections, boosting our important memories.

Sleep is vital for memory in other ways, too. It appears the hippocampus replays the day's activities as we sleep. Indeed, in deep sleep, sleepwalkers literally get up and repeat what they have done during the day.

You may well be shrugging here. Surely we've learned everything we need by now? It's not like the first day at a new school with a zillion names to remember and a ton of learning to do. Up to a point that may be true. Clearly the younger you are, the more you need to learn, hence all that slow-wave sleep. But these days we are working longer than ever, and we want to stay sharp. There's evidence that slow waves may be induced in the brain by two types of gadgets, and research published in the journal *Neuron* in 2013 has shown that stimulating these waves did improve memory.

You can now buy a special type of music that has the right low frequencies to stimulate slow brainwaves – often called brainwave music – and download it into your phone to listen to via headphones or quietly on your iPod speakers overnight.

A type of therapy called Transcranial Magnetic Stimulation (TMS) uses magnetic waves to induce slow brainwaves, and is approved by the US Food and Drug Administration as a treatment for depression, which, as we know, affects sleep and vice versa. Home TMS devices may be used in future to boost slow brainwaves during sleep.

Are You a Lark or an Owl?

The division of people into larks and owls is well known, but it's only recently been discovered that this is down to a specific gene, which comes in two types: the 'lark' gene and the 'owl' gene.

Each of us has two copies of the sleep gene. If both are lark genes, you'll be one of the 10 per cent of people who wake early and perky. Two owl genes will mean you find it hard to wake and are happiest after dark, but if you have one of each type, you'll join the 50 per cent of people who are somewhere in the middle. Larks may be the perky souls at the 7 a.m. yoga class, but they tire earlier and they cope less well with sleep deprivation than owls.

How Much Sleep Do You Need?

A 2013 study published in the *European Journal of Preventive Cardiology* found that healthy people who slept seven or more hours a night were 65 per cent less likely to develop heart disease and 67 per cent less likely to die from it. Remember that heart disease is the number one killer of post-menopausal women, so aim for seven hours as a bare minimum.

You're not getting enough if:

- You feel drowsy during the morning or on the train, or during vital meetings you find yourself desperately battling the urge to nod, snore and drool. Sexy!
- You fall asleep at night almost before your weary head hits the pillow. Non-sleep-deprived people take around fifteen minutes to nod off.

Your Skinny Sleep

We know that high cortisol messes with our metabolism, right? If you get an average of six hours' sleep – you thought that was pretty good, eh? – you are a staggering 27 per cent more likely to be overweight than if you sleep seven to nine hours. And if you get only five hours' sleep, you are 73 per cent more likely to be overweight. In other words, sleep makes you skinny, and tiredness makes you fat.

When you mess with your body clock, this causes changes to genes in the liver, which control the breakdown of fat and glucose, so you lay down fat even if you don't eat more. And the results of lack of sleep show on your body faster than you might imagine.

In a study of sleep, metabolism, appetite and weight at the University of Colorado, it was found that even a few nights of skimped sleep were enough to cause a 2 lb weight gain. The volunteers were kept up until midnight and only allowed to sleep for five hours, and even though their metabolism went up when they were sleep-deprived, they were hungrier, so ate more and craved more high-calorie food. Also, they ate more at night and tended to skip breakfast.

Lack of sleep has the following detrimental effects:

- It increases your hunger hormone ghrelin, which tends to rise in mid-life anyway. Its also triggers fat storage.

- It also makes less leptin, the fullness hormone that tells your body to stop eating and start burning energy.
- After six days of four-hour sleeps, leptin levels start to send signals that your body is facing a famine, making your body desperate for food.
- You may notice you struggle to wake up in the winter. That's because your body wants you to sleep more so that you produce more leptin to tell the body to burn fat gained during the summer. If you don't sleep, that fat sticks around.
- Your body makes more cortisol, which can increase your appetite and dump fat around your middle.
- After just one night of four hours' sleep, your brain's reward centres react more strongly to unhealthy, fatty, sugary food, and the area responsible for self-control doesn't work properly. In other words, cake, chips and mayo become totally irresistible.
- It also affects the way your thyroid works. After six days of four hours' sleep, your levels of thyroid-stimulating hormone fall by more than 30 per cent. Low thyroid activity means we burn less fat.

But there's another surprising way sleep makes you skinny. Sleep actually burns calories – much more than when you are sitting around watching TV or reading. REM sleep is when you dream, and when you are dreaming, your brain is wildly active, burning glucose – even more so than when you are awake. But to get the real benefits of REM sleep, we need to go through five sleep cycles, which takes about seven hours. If we only get six hours' sleep, guess what: we don't get enough vital calorie-burning REM sleep.

What Happens When You Sleep

Every 60–100 minutes we go through four stages of sleep:

Stage 1

Aaah . . . bliss! You are dozing off. You are relaxed. Your heart rate falls. You start to produce very slow brainwaves. This takes only around 5–10 minutes.

Stage 2

You are sleeping, but only lightly. Your body temperature is starting to drop, and your brain produces bursts of rapid, rhythmic brainwave activity. This takes around 20 minutes

Stage 3

Your brain starts producing deep slow brainwaves known as 'delta waves' and you start to transition to . . .

Stage 4

Deep sleep. It's really, really hard to wake up now. If you sleepwalk, it will happen at this stage, which lasts for around 30 minutes.

After deep sleep, we go back to Stage 2 and Stage 3, and then enter . . .

Stage 5

REM (rapid-eye movement) sleep. Now your muscles are very relaxed, so your body doesn't move, but your eyes dart about, your breathing speeds up and your brain goes crazy. The first episode of REM takes only a few minutes, but each time you go through all the stages of sleep it gets longer. By the time you've gone through five cycles, which takes around seven hours, it can last up to an hour. That's an hour of fabulous, no-effort fat burning.

Light Fantastic

Fascinating new research indicates that, as you age, changes to your eyes can make your body clock go crazy. What happens is, the clear lens covering our eyes tends to yellow and our pupils shrink. This combination acts like a pair of sunglasses we can't take off, reducing the amount of sunlight that gets through the lens to regulate the body's internal clock. And the more yellowing of the lens, the more likely you are to sleep badly.

When your pupils are large and your lens clear, light easily passes through to photoreceptor cells at the back of your eye. These transmit messages to the brain to regulate the amount of melatonin you secrete in the evening to make you sleepy, and cortisol in the morning to wake you up.

Melatonin is also a super-antioxidant, which is vital for preventing disease; it lifts your mood and regulates your sleep/wake cycles. The most important kind of light is blue light, which is increasingly filtered out by your eye's ageing lens. A study in *The British Journal of Ophthalmology* found that by the age of forty-five, your photoreceptors may only get half of the light they need to make your sleep/wake cycle work properly. By age fifty-five, we get only 37 per cent. This means it's harder for older women to produce enough melatonin, which affects our sleep, memory and mood. And so that glorious high from a sunny day becomes ever more elusive.

What Can You Do to Get Your Vital Light Fix?

We evolved to spend most of our time outdoors. So get out in the day when natural light is at its strongest – ideally in the morning and at midday. Artificial lights are not only up to 10,000 times dimmer than sunlight, they are the wrong colour light to stimulate the brain. Drink your morning coffee in the garden, walk to work, and work out outdoors instead of at the gym as often as you can. If you have to be indoors, use daylight-simulating bulbs in your home and sit by a window. In the winter, you might want to invest in a special lightbox developed to simulate bright summer light and aimed at sufferers of Seasonal Affective Disorder (a type of winter depression that causes tiredness, clumsiness, indecisiveness and low mood). Light intensity is measured in units of lux.

Ordinary light bulbs only emit around 200–500 lux. To treat SAD you need a light source with at least 2,500 lux and ideally around 10,000 lux. Treatment normally starts in autumn, before symptoms set in. With the most powerful boxes you may only need around half an hour's exposure a day, compared to up to three hours with less. You can work, read or eat your breakfast while in front of the box.

Supercharge Your Sleep

There are lots of ways to help us sleep better, no matter what our genetic programming. Apart from the obvious – don't drink espressos after 3 p.m., don't drink lots of alcohol or stay up until 3 a.m. playing video games on brightly lit screens – try some of the following:

- Take a bath before bed. This is not just to relax you; cooling the body triggers sleep, and the best way to ensure cooling is to get warmed up first! A hot foot bath may be a substitute for a full body bath.

- Heating the skin on your stomach or chest may help you fall asleep more quickly. A hot water bottle should do the trick.
- When you wake up, set your sleep cycle by getting a few minutes of bright natural light on your face as a soon as you can and for at least thirty minutes. Even a cloudy day is many, many times brighter than an artificially lit room.
- Just do it. Most of us don't get enough sleep. If we go to bed earlier, it's likely we will fall asleep and get the sleep we need, deserve and, let's face it, enjoy.

Eat to Sleep

Now you know why sleep is crucial to your health, happiness and hormones, here's how to get more of it. As you've seen, melatonin is a powerful sleep aid. Supplements are not available over the counter in the UK, though they can be bought in the US. However, these foods contain natural melatonin.

- Top of the list of melatonin-rich foods is a type of tart cherry called a Montmorency cherry. A recent study found that drinking concentrated cherry juice can improve sleep quality and duration.
- Walnuts
- Sunflower seeds
- Oats

Other Sleep Foods to Try

- Kiwi fruit is rich in magnesium, vitamin C, folic acid and serotonin, which act to relax muscles and calm nerve activity. A recent study revealed that eating two kiwi fruit an hour before bedtime helped people fall asleep significantly faster, and that they slept longer and better.
- Bananas contain potassium and magnesium, which are natural muscle relaxants. They also contain the amino acid L-tryptophan, which gets converted to 5-HTP in the brain. The 5-HTP in turn is converted to serotonin (a relaxing neurotransmitter) and melatonin.
- Milk also contains L-tryptophan, and is high in calcium, which promotes sleep.
- Turkey is particularly high in L-tryptophan, which can also be found in protein foods such as chicken, eggs, fish and beans. But you need to eat some carbs with these animal proteins, otherwise another amino acid they contain, tyrosine, will keep you awake.
- Serotonin is also produced when we eat carbohydrates. You can also increase serotonin by taking exercise, practising yoga and meditation, and eating foods that contains the building blocks for serotonin, such as chicken, seafood, fish, eggs and soya products.

- If you can't sleep, eating a small amount of rice or pasta in the evening may help by gently spiking insulin, which then reduces, leaving you sleepy.

Sleep Saboteurs

- Caffeine – found in coffee and tea. We all know it can make us jittery and wakeful. Cut it out after noon if you can't sleep.
- Drinking seriously messes with your sleep cycle. Alcohol drunk within an hour of bedtime disrupts the second half of your sleep cycle – yes, the bit that keeps you thin. Studies show that even alcohol drunk up to six hours before bed can keep you awake. This is long after it has left your bloodstream, which suggests that alcohol has a long-term effect on your body's sleep cycle. So have a cocktail or a glass of wine, by all means, but the more you drink, the less you'll sleep.
- Fatty foods. New studies show that eating a high-fat diet disturbs your sleep. Too much fat reduces brain sensitivity to orexin, a brain chemical important in stabilizing sleep and wake states.
- The perfect pre-sleep meal? Try turkey and a little wholegrain rice with green vegetables. Follow with a fruit salad, including bananas and kiwi fruit with yoghurt, eaten no later than three hours before bedtime. Late eating interferes with your deep 'skinny sleep'. If you eat well at supper, you

shouldn't be hungry, but if you are, have a small snack of protein and carbs an hour before bed. Good choices include egg on toast, or a little cheese on oatcakes, or a banana and some nuts.

Take Control!

For great sleep you need to learn some healthy sleep habits. A regular sleep schedule, where you go to bed and wake up at the same time, is proven to help you sleep. But a pre-sleep schedule is also vital. Here's your countdown to a great night:

- **Six hours before bed** – have your last alcoholic drink. OK, that may be unreasonable if you are at dinner or a party, but remember, every drink you have later than this can stymie sleep.
- **Four hours before bed** – exercise. A workout can leave you healthily tired, but don't exercise later than three hours before bed, to allow your body time to cool down, which is a natural sleep trigger. You can do yoga and stretches before bedtime, as these help you relax.
- **Three hours before bed** – take a hot bath or shower to heat your body and then let it cool.
- **Two hours before bed** – turn off your screens. The light from TVs, tablets, laptops and even your phone, confuses your brain, so it produces up to 22 per cent less melatonin after only two

hours of screen time. Non-backlit screens such as Kindles are OK.

- **Ninety minutes before bed** – dim your lights. Low light triggers melatonin. Sleep in a dark, quiet room.
- **One hour before bed** – open a window or turn off the heating in your bedroom. A cool (not cold) room will stimulate sleep and help keep night sweats at bay. Wear socks to keep your core temperature stable.
- **Thirty minutes before bed** – open a book. Remember, reading something absorbing can reduce stress levels by more than two-thirds in just six minutes!

'I refuse to admit that I am more than fifty-two, even if that makes my children illegitimate.'
Nancy Astor

6. Take Control: Metabolism

The Secret of Timing Your Meals for a Leaner Body Without Dieting

We love to eat! Hell, unless you met your man within the last six weeks, eating is better than sex. And luckily we all get to do it several times a day. Yippee. But lots of us have a love/hate relationship with food. We love the taste, we hate being hungry (soooo grumpy-making), we love to be whisked out to dinner by our man, or to have a laughter-filled supper with a girlfriend or two. But on the other hand, we worry about food making us fat.

We feel guilty about how healthy our diet is, and know the calorific value of everything from an egg to a doughnut. It shouldn't be this way, but we'll bet you are nodding away in agreement. You absolutely do not have to be thin to be healthy. In fact, weight gain in mid-life is natural, and provided you stay active and keep away from processed and junk food, a bit of plumpness, right up at the top of the BMI range, and even above, doesn't harm your health and may even be linked to longer life (you can work out your BMI using free online calculators).

On the other hand, most of you probably still want to fit into your clothes and to recognize your body in the mirror. You might find you struggle with inexorably rising weight as the years go by, and that the diets you try just don't seem to work the way they used to when you were young. You know from previous chapters that hormonal changes can cause weight gain, even if you don't change the way you eat, and they also affect our body shape. Before the menopause, if your hormones are healthy, oestrogen directs fat to your hips and thighs, where it's locked in safely to provide fuel for pregnancy. It's why it's so hard for most of us to lose weight from our hips when we are younger. But when oestrogen levels drop, fat is released from those areas and instead goes to our belly, and to a lesser extent to our arms, where it is similarly locked in. This might be to help us produce bone-preserving oestrogen from fat cells after the menopause – our bodies are smart and don't do things for no reason – but few of us enjoy this particular change! So what can you do?

Look, we don't want you to stop eating, even if was possible. Crazy, calorie-controlled diets don't work. They just make *you* crazy. Research shows that dieting makes the brain more sensitive to stress – yes, more of that horrible cortisol – and more easily tempted by high-fat, high-calorie treats. Levels of hunger hormones soar and the hormones that make you feel full fall. These brain changes last long after the diet is over – up to a year – and seem to be the link to post-diet bingeing. Up to 98 per cent of women who lose weight on calorie-controlled diets regain every last pound – and often add a few extra.

We want you to love your food, eat well, go out and have fun, and still stay well and look good. And what we want to tell you is that when it comes to keeping your weight under control, calories really don't count. I know that sounds contrary to everything you've ever heard, but it's true. The type of food you eat and the time you eat it actually matters much more. Yes, you don't want to stuff yourself silly, but you can eat and enjoy food and stay healthy, as long as you eat *the right stuff at the right time*.

But first, some bad news. We honestly hate to break this to you, but your metabolic rate – the speed with which you burn off energy from food – is getting slower as you age. It actually starts to slow down from the age of twenty. We know! Twenty! By the time you are forty, it has fallen by about 10 per cent, and it keeps right on dropping. What's more, your hunger hormones start working overtime, especially if you are coming up to, or are in, the menopause.

Yup. You need less food, yet you want to eat more food. But don't panic. There are ways to get your metabolism all revved up, and even to turn those hunger hormones right down – and the really great news is, you can literally do this in your sleep. A quick note. Exercise is really important if you want your metabolic rate to be on your side. We promise we are going to talk about that a bit later, but right now we're concentrating on food.

You know from previous chapters about how sleep and stress affect your hormones, and that these changes affect your appetite and metabolism. Now new research shows that it's not just *what* you eat, but *when* you eat that affects how much energy you store as fat. By the way, if you really want to lose some weight quickly, at the end of the book you'll find our unique, no-calories-involved, hormone-balancing fat-loss plan, as devised by Dr Daniel Sister. But hang on, don't skip to there quite yet! We're about to unveil the tricks that will help you boost your metabolism, stop you eating when you aren't really hungry, and keep your body vibrant and at a healthy weight for ever.

Start as You Mean to Go On

Remember when your mother told you, 'Don't skip breakfast, eat regular meals and don't snack late at night . . . ? Well, she was right. And she wasn't even a scientist.

New research indicates you could lose weight without dieting, simply by condensing your meals into a regular time span of around eight hours. Basically, instead of starving by day, you slim as you sleep. How? In experiments on mice (yes, we know you aren't a mouse, but bear with us) one group of rodents was given a very high-fat, high-calorie diet – the equivalent of deep-pan pizza, chips and cheesecake, which they ate over an eight-hour period, during the time they were normally active (day for us, night for them). They then didn't eat for sixteen hours, which included their sleep time. In human terms, this sort of timing is the equivalent of having your last meal at 5 p.m., and eating your breakfast at 9 a.m.

like intermittent fasting

Meanwhile, a second group of mice were given exactly the same food, with exactly the same amount of calories, but this time they were allowed to eat around the clock.

So what happened to those gluttonous mice, stuffed full of delicious, fattening treats all day? The group of mice who ate day and night became, as you might imagine, obese. They also developed high cholesterol, high blood sugar and fatty liver disease. But what about the first group? The ones who stopped eating for sixteen hours?

Scientists were amazed because these mice did not gain weight. Compared to the snackers, they were a staggering 28 per cent thinner. And not only that, they showed hardly any signs of inflammation or liver disease, and their cholesterol and blood sugar levels were the same as those of mice on a healthy diet. What's more, when put on a mouse treadmill (yes, they do have them), they had more endurance and the best motor control of all the mice, including mice on a natural low-fat diet. Hell, these rodents were supermice! But why did this happen? It seems that as the mice snoozed on an empty stomach, enzymes in their teeny livers start to break down cholesterol. And a type of fat called 'brown fat' became more active, thus speeding up their metabolism. Yup, the metabolisms of the fasting mice actually increased. As they slept, the mice livers were burning fat. Lots of fat!

The Body Clock Connection

But does any of this apply to humans? Yes, the evidence indicates that it does. You have an internal clock called a circadian rhythm. This is hormonally driven and has effects on all aspects of your body's functions. For example, your blood pressure rises between 8 a.m. and noon and is lowest at midnight. Your heartbeat follows an internal clock, too, and so, says new research, does your appetite and your ability to burn fat. Your body really hates getting out of whack with this clock – as anyone who has felt like death due to jet lag will know.

It seems we need to rest our digestive systems overnight for optimum health and maximum fat burning. Late-night eating seems to make you fatter and sicker. Shift workers are fatter than people who work regular daytime hours; they are also more likely to be diabetic and to have high cholesterol. Why? During the day, your body – more specifically your brain and muscles – uses some of the calories you eat for fuel, and stores the rest in your liver in the form of glycogen. At night that glycogen gets turned into glucose and is released into your bloodstream, so your blood sugar levels stay steady while you sleep. Once the stored glycogen is gone, your liver starts burning fat cells for energy. Yes, you read that right, if your body isn't full of sugar, you burn fat while you sleep.

The catch? It takes a few hours for your body to use up those glycogen stores. So if you eat right up until you go to bed and have a full stomach at midnight, then eat breakfast at 7 a.m., your body may never get the opportunity to burn any fat before you start reloading your glycogen stores.

It doesn't help that you're also likely to overeat when you're up late. Night owls consume an average of 248 calories more per day than those who go to bed earlier, and most of those extra calories rack up after 8 p.m.

So how long should you 'fast' overnight? It is possible that sixteen hours is optimum, but let's face it, for most of us it's not practical, or sociable, to do this every day. There's no point in being such a fanatic that you can't have dinner with friends, or share a meal with your man at the end of the working day. In fact, cutting back on your social life is really unhealthy. But it seems reasonable to try to go twelve hours without eating overnight as often as you can.

As it's unhealthy to skip breakfast, the easiest, healthiest plan seems to be to try to finish eating relatively early. So if you finish dinner at 8 p.m., you can then eat breakfast at 8 a.m. Remember, that 8 p.m. curfew includes stopping drinking wine, juice and milk – anything that adds sugar and calories to your body. Water is fine. And if you can eat a light supper and get an early night a couple of times a week, giving yourself a fourteen- to sixteen-hour eating break, that's a big bonus.

The huge benefit of this way of eating is that you don't have to starve and you don't have to count calories. In fact, you can eat what you like, but of course, if you want to reap the real benefits, stick to the kind of healthy, hormone-balancing, natural foods we recommend in the next chapter.

When it comes to fasting, you've probably heard about intermittent fasting, or the 5:2 diet, where you eat almost nothing – just 500 calories – for two or three days a week. It's claimed that this not only keeps you thin, but also makes you healthier, reducing levels of ageing hormones and even making you live longer. It's extremely trendy, but like so many things, the much-touted benefits are the results of trials on men, and there's evidence that this kind of semi-starvation doesn't benefit women hormonally, especially if you haven't yet hit the menopause. It may even affect women's production of the hormone insulin, making them have worse blood sugar control, not better. It may stress the body, too, causing cortisol to rise and increasing peptides in the brain that boost appetite and alertness, which might seem like a good thing, but in women can trigger insomnia – and we now know how important sleep is.

To add to the problems, new evidence shows that calorie restriction doesn't increase lifespan in our nearest relatives, apes, as we used to think it did. If you are pre-menopausal, and that includes the peri-menopausal period, and do intermittent fasting, you could be causing hormonal havoc in your body.

We've talked to women who have tried intermittent fasting and found it has caused sleeplessness, anxiety and sometimes stopped their periods – all signs of hormonal havoc. The theory is that fasting messes with hypocretin neurons. These are neurons in the brain that are vital for both healthy appetite and healthy sleep. If they think we are starving, they make us wakeful – it's an evolutionary thing, so that we keep looking for food.

But there are other problems associated with skipping meals. In a 2007 study reported in the *American Journal of Clinical Nutrition*, it was reported, 'After three weeks of alternate day fasting, women but not men had an increase in the area under the glucose curve.' Huh? Well, what this means is that the more they fasted, the worse their blood sugar control got. As the study reported, 'This unfavorable effect on glucose tolerance in women, accompanied by an apparent lack of an effect on insulin sensitivity, suggests that short-term ADF may be more beneficial in men than in women in reducing type 2 diabetes risk.' In other words, alternate day fasting could make women more at risk of diabetes! This does not mean you shouldn't do it at all, but we think doing it before the menopause may be risky, and even afterwards it could raise your stress and hunger hormones.

Also, let's face it, hunger is no fun. It makes us miserable, bad-tempered, weak and tired, and few of us can fight it for long. It's nearly impossible to exercise on days when you don't eat, and also, most of us like to eat in a social way, and don't want to become a hermit several days a week for the rest of our lives. Because to get any benefits out of intermittent fasting, you do have to keep it up for ever. Good luck with that, normal people!

Leah tried fasting pre-menopause and found that not only was she a complete witch on 500 calories, but she became totally obsessed with food, and on her 'eating days' she found herself eating giant spoonfuls of cheesecake direct from the fridge. Not a pretty sight. 'I felt possessed,' she says. I don't even like cheesecake!'

By doing your 'fasting' mostly at night, when you don't even notice it and you don't feel hungry, you can get into fat-burning mode, change your hormone balance for the better and still eat without worrying about calorie restriction, which, as we have seen, can be horrible for some women's health. We think this 'flexi-fasting' has to be a better plan for us mere mortals.

Breakfast Like a King

OK, you had your supper early, slept well, and now it is morning and you are S-T-A-R-V-I-N-G.

The tempting thing when you want to stay slim or lose weight is to skip breakfast and make do with a dose of caffeine instead. Bad move! Didn't your mama tell you that eating breakfast kick-starts your metabolism? It's true! Breakfast boosts your metabolism by up to 10 per cent. And that's just part of the story. Breakfast is the meal that most effectively suppresses the hunger hormone, ghrelin, while the morning's high cortisol levels trigger fat and calorie burning.

Eating breakfast also sends a signal to your body clock that you are up and ready for action, which gets that metabolism revving. Indeed, we are programmed by nature to eat more in the morning and less as the day goes on.

Studies show that food eaten until midday is more filling and if we eat well in the morning, this will ensure we are less hungry during the rest of the day. Food eaten in the evening is less filling, so it triggers us to want to eat more, and more often. For decades Dr Sister has told his patients that they can eat pretty much anything they want for breakfast, including chocolate croissants – well, he is French – and keep their weight steady.

And a recent study has proved his advice to be absolutely correct. In an Israeli study, people were put on a low-carb diet with the same overall calories, but while some stuck to a 300-calorie breakfast allowance, others were given a massive 600-calorie breakfast, including a fry-up, and (we love this!) chocolate cake. After sixteen weeks, both groups had lost a respectable 33 lbs per person. But by thirty-two weeks, the strict, small-breakfast group had regained 22 lbs – oops! – while the big break-fasters lost another 15 lbs each, ending up a staggering 48 lbs lighter. Why?

Partly, it seems, the lucky breakfast gorgers just didn't feel as hungry, and they didn't have cravings so they stuck to their diets much more effectively. But also, we have seen that food timing makes a difference to how we use energy. Obviously, you don't have to start eating cake every day – in fact, we don't recommend it – but equally, don't deny yourself. Some people just want lots of fruit for breakfast, which is fine. But for optimum hunger-taming, get some protein in there somewhere – people who eat eggs for breakfast are less hungry all day. Don't like eggs? Try some yoghurt, maybe some nuts, avocado on rye, smoked salmon, or go continental with meat and cheese.

When and What Should You Eat?

Studies indicate the key to a healthy metabolism is to eat regularly and not too late. You can eat three meals or four or even six, as long you don't get too hungry in between, you don't eat too late and your portions aren't too generous. You might find that three meals a day, plus two small, healthy snacks mid-morning and mid-afternoon, help you stay on schedule.

When You've Got Your Timing Right, What Should You Eat to Max Your Metabolism?

We now know that a low-carb, high-protein diet keeps metabolisms revving fastest. Sugar and white processed carbs are your enemy. They fill you full of the hormone insulin, which makes your body store fat. Metabolic rate drops the most in people on a high-carb, low-glycaemic diet, though this diet has benefits in reducing inflammation.

A low-fat diet falls in the middle, but pushes up levels of the hunger hormone leptin, which means keeping weight off could be a problem. You can use super-fat-burning foods and supplements to ensure you eat plenty, but don't gain weight. Here are some of our favourites:

- **Oily fish** – Omega-3 fats, the type found in fish, such as salmon, mackerel and fresh tuna, may boost metabolism. Supplements of fish oils can reduce body fat, increase lean muscle and reduce cortisol, the stress hormone that makes us lay down fat.
- **Fibre** – Fruits, vegetables and whole grains take longer to digest because the body has to work harder to break down the fibre. The type of fibre in fruit and vegetables is particularly effective at reducing your appetite. A nice extra? Fibre also helps balance your hormones by helping your

body excrete waste oestrogen, possibly reducing your risk of breast cancer and fibroids.

- **Spice** – Spicy food and curries can increase metabolism for hours after eating. An ingredient called capsaicin increases body temperature, which burns calories.
- **Green tea and caffeine** – Yes, that lovely coffee can also increase your calorie burn, while green tea is rich in antioxidants.
- **Protein** – It takes over three times as much energy to digest protein as fat, so for every 100 calories of protein you eat, 27 calories will be required simply to digest it. Also, eating more protein can reduce the number of calories the average person consumes by around 450 per day. This is because protein boosts levels of a hunger-fighting hormone known as peptide YY (PYY). Simply eating more protein makes your body produce more natural PYY, so you feel fuller and less hungry.
- **Dairy foods** – They aren't for everyone, but if you can digest them, the combination of calcium and a substance called CLA (conjugated linoleic acid) may push up your metabolic rate. Women who eat dairy, such as yoghurt, and even full-fat cheese, tend to be slimmer. And fatty acids found in dairy fats can reduce the risk of diabetes.
- **Nuts** – These are highly nutritious, boost your serotonin levels and rev up your metabolism by

up to 11 per cent. Nuts don't seem to be digested fully by the body, and they stimulate the production of cholecystokinin (CCK), which is a hormone that not only turns down the dial on your appetite, but also slows down the rate at which your stomach empties. Eating nuts is associated with a slimmer body, and despite the fear that nuts are fatty and high in calories, people who add raw nuts to their diet don't normally gain weight. In a 2005 study at the University of California, it was found that women produced more CKK in response to nut oils such as walnut oil and pine-nut oil, and that low-fat meals, or even meals with vegetable oils, were not as satisfying as ones containing nut oils.

- **Dark chocolate** – We love you, so we'll leave you with the news that people who eat antioxidant-rich, low-sugar dark chocolate found their appetites reduced for salty, sweet and fatty foods afterwards.
- **Water** – Drinking just two extra glasses of water per day can boost your metabolism by 30 per cent and increase your concentration levels, too. Most of us are slightly dehydrated anyway, which suppresses our metabolic rate, so those extra glasses are really just bringing our metabolic machinery back to optimal function, and accelerating fat loss in the process.

Take Control of Your Portion Size

Guess what? You're not hungry, you just think you are. This is absolutely true, and we have the science to prove it. Here's how to unthink your hunger, eat less and feel satisfied.

It's horribly easy to gain fat in mid-life. We know that; we understand and we know that for health and vanity reasons (OK, especially for getting-into-clothes reasons) you don't want to pile on the pounds as you age. But we also know it's important not to get hungry, because this raises our stress hormone cortisol, which in turn triggers our brain to crave food.

And not just any food, but unhealthy, sugary, fatty, crisps-chips-and-cake junk food. We've given you lots of information about how to eat plenty of food without gaining weight. You know that cutting down on carbs, especially starchy, white carbs, is important. You know that sleeping more and stressing less is important. But hunger truly isn't just a matter of what we do or don't eat. It's much more complicated than that. How our food looks and, vitally, what we think and believe about food plays a huge role in how hungry we are. For example, in a 2008 study at the Department of Food Science at Purdue University (the source, by the way, of the studies from which the following tips have been drawn) people were given a drink or a solid snack (like a cube of jelly), and before they consumed it they were told one of four things would happen:

- Some people given the liquid were told it would stay a liquid once it was swallowed.
- Others were told it would become solid once it was swallowed.
- Of those given a solid, some were told it would remain solid.
- Others were told it would turn into a liquid in their stomach.

In fact, both the liquid and solids ended up as liquid in the stomach. What happens next is really interesting. Those who were told that the liquid or solid would remain solid after it was swallowed reported feeling more full. So far, so unsurprising. But this fullness wasn't just an illusion in the stomach. It affected the body, the brain and the hormonal system. The women who thought their stomachs were full produced less of the hunger hormone ghrelin and their stomachs emptied more slowly than those of the people who believed their stomach contained liquid. Those who believed they'd only had liquid ate more later in the day – a whopping 400 calories more – than those who thought they'd eaten something solid. Incredible, eh? The truth is, if we think something will fill us up, it will.

So how can you use this knowledge that the brain tricks the body into keeping you lean? Here are ten cunning ways to eat less, while feeling fuller:

1. **USE SMALLER PLATES** (and bowls and cutlery). People laughed when it was revealed that Elizabeth Hurley attributed her fabulous body to 'eating off a tiny plate and using small cutlery', but

hey, just look at her. And she's right. Portion sizes have soared over the decades. In one cookbook, the serving sizes for main courses were sometimes 62 per cent bigger in the 2006 edition than in the original 1920 edition. No wonder we're getting bigger, too. Researchers have shown that if you shrink the diameter of your plate from 30 cm to 25 cm, you will reduce the amount you eat. And it could easily be more. In one study those who spooned ice cream into small bowls ate 31 per cent less than those with big bowls, yet, crucially, felt just as full.

2. **GET SOME BLUE PLATES**. People eat less when their food contrasts with the colour of their plates, presumably because it's easier to see just how much you are eating. In a study, people eating white pasta in a cream sauce off a white plate ate 22 per cent more than people who were given a red plate. Blue is a good idea because no food is a true blue, and it's a colour that doesn't stimulate appetite. On the other hand, if you want to eat more green vegetables, eat from a green plate.

3. **DISH OUT SMALLER PORTIONS ON PURPOSE**. People eat 92 per cent of what they serve themselves – however much they put on their plate. We suggest a serving size of around the amount of food you could fit into your cupped hands. Then wait for three hours before you eat again.

4. **NEVER EAT OUT OF THE PACKET**.
Our habit of mindless eating means we'll keep
eating if we don't recognize how much of a food
equals a portion. So we'll eat far more if we're
eating biscuits out of the packet or even grapes
out of the bag. Buy smaller packets and bags, take
out the amount you want to eat, and no more,
and serve it in one of your small blue bowls.

5. **KEEP YOUR TRIGGER FOODS OUT
OF THE KITCHEN**. Hey, come on, we bet
you have at least one. Leah can't leave prawn
crackers alone, Susie is unstoppable when she
gets her hands on pretzels. So we don't buy them.
Problem solved. The same goes for all foods you
don't want to eat for health or dress-size reasons.
If it's not there, you can't eat it.

6. **DON'T BUY PROCESSED FOODS
WITH A LOW-FAT LABEL**. People eat up
to 23 per cent more of food that's labelled low
fat. Plus, these low-fat foods are often packed
with salt or sugar to 'improve the flavour'.
Though frankly, we think they still taste horrible.

7. **IN RESTAURANTS ASK FOR A
DOGGY BAG BEFORE YOU START
EATING**. Given the humungous portions in
restaurants today (we sometimes feel nostalgic
for nouvelle cuisine, to be honest), we like to
order a starter as a main course with extra vegetables or salad. But if you can't resist a main

course and it looks like a hefty serving, ask your waiter to bag up half of it before you start. It's likely you'll never feel hungry enough to eat it and, of course, you already wave away the bread basket – don't you?

8. **SLOW DOWN**. People who are effortlessly thin chew more than people who aren't. The most effective way to achieve this is to start eating at your normal pace, then consciously slow down your chewing rate halfway through your meal. That way, you may never want to finish it.

9. **EAT WITHOUT DISTRACTIONS**. The TV, a magazine, the radio are all big no-nos. Eating with people is fine, of course, but don't get so carried away that you forget about what you are eating. Think about your food, make a decision to savour the taste and note how you feel as you eat it. You will enjoy it more, eat less and enjoy your reflection more, too.

10. **COOK FOR PLEASURE AS MUCH AS HEALTH**. The better your food tastes, the less deprived you will feel. Skinny people tend not to force down food they don't like.

11. **DON'T EAT WHITE**. Cut out nearly all white foods – flour, bread, sugar, rice. Of course, some whites do you good, such as lean turkey and chicken, and natural live yoghurt. If we spot you eating the odd slice of birthday cake and croissants on holiday, we won't tell if you don't . . .

Take Control!

- Eat regular meals.
- Try to go twelve hours overnight without eating or drinking anything except water as often as you can.
- Go sixteen hours without eating overnight once or twice a week, providing you can still sleep well.
- Always eat breakfast (cake is optional).
- Eat metabolism-boosting foods, especially protein.
- Drink plenty of water.

'Maybe it's true that life begins at fifty . . . but everything else starts to wear out, fall out, or spread out.'
Phyllis Diller, American comedian

7. Take Control: Eat yourself YOUNG

Youth Food!

In the previous chapter we told you about foods that help you stay slim, foods that help your hormones and foods that rev up your metabolism – but this chapter is all about the sheer pleasure of health. These are our favourite foods to make you feel and look utterly fabulous. Base your diet on these superfoods and they'll help you turn back the clock.

A diet rich in vitamins, amino acids and antioxidants is absolutely key to slowing and reversing ageing. Remember those telomeres, the scary cell tails of doom? These little tips on chromosomes shorten as we age, but an enzyme called telomerase can protect your telomeres, and telomerase is increased in women with high intakes of vitamins D, E and C.

Research published in the March 2012 issue of the journal *PLOS ONE* showed that eating just three portions of fruit and vegetables a day makes you prettier. The study looked at what people ate and at their skin tone. If you eat fruit and veg, your skin takes on yellow and red pigments from them, which makes you rosy and glowing. Positively peachy, in fact.

Those who had more of these pigments in their diet were voted more gorgeous than their pasty, veg-hating counterparts. You see, plants are full of nutrients that aren't just minerals and vitamins. They include things that give them their colour and taste, such as carotenoids, flavonoids and isoflavonoids. They are powerful anti-oxidants, which protect your DNA, turn off inflammation and keep your immune system firing as though you were years younger. They can even protect your skin against sunburn and ageing.

Some scientists believe that if you cut out three servings of refined carbs and replaced them with fruit, vegetables, nuts and beans, you could cut diet-related disease rates by half. So add these gorgeous superfoods to your shopping list:

SUPERFOOD SHOPPING LIST

SPINACH AND KALE	Have been proven to help improve skin hydration and elasticity. How? Dark, leafy greens contain lots of antioxidants called 'lutein' and beta-carotene, which are known to improve skin elasticity and firmness. (These are Leah's favourite vegetables. She says, 'They take just a few minutes to cook, so I always keep bags of pre-prepared spinach and kale to throw into casseroles or simply serve steamed and lightly buttered. Butter not only makes them utterly delicious but fat helps your body absorb carotenes'.)

TURKEY	Not just a holiday treat any more, but of course make sure it's organic. The carnosine in white Turkey meat is now known to slow the deterioration of collagen in the skin. Turkey is also a source of phenylalanine, and studies show phenylalanine can be as effective against depression as taking anti-depressants.
RED AND YELLOW PEPPERS	As well as being considered superfoods for the skin because of their high antioxidant properties, peppers are now known to offer extra UV protection, according to research at the University of Arizona. Amazing news for us sun lovers.
OLIVES	A skin-boosting snack – the more olives you eat, the less wrinkled your skin appears, according to research by Monash University in Australia. Thank you, Australians, for providing us with this research, as we do love our olives.
OLIVE OIL	For those that don't like olives. Have at least one tablespoon a day. Olive oil is 'good fat,' as it contains heart-healthy omega-3s, which improve your circulation leaving the skin rosy and supple.
RASPBERRIES	Contain ellagic acid, which is known to help protect collagen. Studies also show raspberry extract can inhibit the inflammation response that causes some skin cancers.

BANANAS Are not fattening, it's a myth. Bananas are slightly higher in energy than other fruits but the calories come mainly from carbohydrate; excellent for refuelling before, during or after exercise. Bananas are also jam-packed with potassium that helps lower blood pressure and vitamin B6 for healthy skin and hair. Says Susie, 'I always have them before I work out or as a pick-me-up after a long day.'

BRAZIL NUTS Like other nuts, Brazils are generally full of essential vitamins, minerals and fibre. Recent studies suggest that eating a small handful of nuts four times a week can help reduce heart disease and satisfy food cravings. Brazil nuts are one of the few good sources of selenium that may help protect against cancer, depression and Alzheimer's disease. Anything that makes you less depressed and protects you against all the nasties is going to make you appear younger and happier.

WATERMELON Great for a hydrated, soft complexion. Watermelon contains lots of vitamin C, potassium and lycopene. These ultimate antioxidants help to regulate the balance of water and nutrients in cells. And new research, published in the *Journal of Nutritional Biochemistry*, suggest that citrulline, a compound found in watermelon, plays a role in heart health. Mice (yes, them again) given watermelon juice had lower cholesterol and clearer arteries than other mice.

BLUEBERRIES — Packed full of flavonoids and polyphenols, which protect against inflammation, blueberries prevent cell-structure damage that can lead to fine lines, wrinkles and loss of skin firmness. They may also protect the brain from ageing.

GREEN TEA — Helps diminish brown spots. We knew green tea was good for you, but this is a great find. Not only is this healthy brew great for your diet and boosting your metabolism, it contains 'catechins,' an effective compound for preventing premature ageing and the effects of sun damage. Green tea is rich in antioxidants that fight off free radical damage.

OILY COLD-WATER FISH: SALMON, SARDINES OR MACKEREL — Naturally contain omega-3 fatty acids, which strengthen skin-cell membranes helping to hydrate the skin and reduce redness and inflammation. They also make your telomeres stay long for longer as they help your body make magic telomerase.

POMEGRANATE — This Middle Eastern fruit is known to combat heart disease, as well as containing three times as many cancer-fighting antioxidants as green tea. It is believed to be particularly effective in warding off prostate cancer and, very possibly, breast cancer. Pomegranates have effective antibacterial properties and have also been shown to alleviate the symptoms of osteoarthritis. Pomegranate has high levels of vitamin C, which is necessary for healthy skin, teeth, bones and connective tissue. What doesn't it do?

COLOUR ME BEAUTIFUL

Fruits and vegetables come in a variety of colours.
By choosing different coloured groups, get the most
benefit from your diet.

GREEN:
Phytochemicals are present in all
green fruits and vegetables. Lutein, found in
deep green veg, can protect your eyes, keeping
cataracts at bay and also increasing the amount of
blue light that gets through to your retinas.
Remember from our chapter on sleep, you normally
absorb less blue light as your eyes yellow with age.
This means you make less melatonin, don't sleep as well,
and don't get that 'Hey! It's a sunny day! I feel amazing!'
boost from sunlight. Lutein can prevent that
happening. Phytochemicals may possibly
reduce the risk of cancerous tumours.
EAT spinach, broccoli, kale, Brussels
sprouts, cauliflower and turnips.

SIMPLY RED:
Lycopene is the main
antioxidant found in red
and pink fruits and vegetables.
It may protect against breast
cancer and cervical cancer.
EAT tomatoes, grapefruit,
watermelons and
papayas.

OANGE/YELLOW:
Carotenoids are natural
antioxidants that are the main
components of beta-carotene, the
substance that makes carrots carroty.
Great for your immune system.
EAT sweet potatoes, corn,
carrots, mangoes, oranges,
pineapples and pears.

BLUE/PURPLE:
Anthocyanin, another type
of phytochemical, is incredibly
potent as an antioxidant and
immunity booster. It helps build
the body's defence mechanism to
fight harmful carcinogens, and
is highly anti-ageing.
EAT blueberries,
blackberries and red
grapes.

WHITE:
Allicin is a phytochemical
that can lower cholesterol
and blood pressure, and
helps you to fight infections.
EAT onions, leeks, garlic,
shallots, pears, green grapes
and cauliflower.

What is a Serving of Fruit or Veg?

Think of one serving of fruit and vegetables as the amount that would fit into the palm of your hand. Not much, eh? You should try to eat five to nine fruits and vegetables each day. Come on, you can do it – especially if you eat fewer biscuits! Here's how.

One serving equals:

- A small glass of 100 per cent freshly squeezed fruit or vegetable juice (¾ cup or 175 ml)
- A medium-sized piece of fruit – an orange, small banana or medium-sized apple
- 1 cup of raw salad leaves
- One medium tomato or seven cherry tomatoes
- ½ cup of cooked vegetables
- ½ cup of cut-up fruit or vegetables as crudités or pudding
- ¼ cup of dried fruit
- ½ cup of cooked beans or peas

Take Control!

- Eat leafy green vegetables.
- Don't be afraid of nuts.

- Eat a rainbow of food colours.
- Stick to portion sizes.

'The secret to staying young is to live honestly, eat slowly and lie about your age.'
  Lucille Ball

8. Take Control: Sex Life

Are You Getting Enough?

Great sex makes you look and feel younger and happier. Do you know what we think is one of the greatest myths about ageing? It's that women over a certain age don't care about sex, don't want sex, don't like sex, worst of all, shouldn't like sex.

We say, 'No to that!' We know that most women in mid-life still want to be passionate, to feel desired and desirable, and to enjoy sex. Yes, sex isn't compulsory at any age, but neither is champagne or Chanel. And great sex definitely makes life better.

A lively libido and a hot sex life keep you feeling young and boost your confidence – perhaps because it's hard to hate your body when it's making you extremely happy on a regular basis. Sex is also a fabulous way to boost your health and wellbeing.

Here's why. When you fall in love (OK, and lust) you produce huge amounts of a neurohormone called beta-phenylethylamine (PEA). PEA boosts the effects of dopamine, a brain chemical that in turn boosts wellbeing and, pleasure, and fires the reward centres of the brain. Norepinephrine is a powerful brain stimulant that creates wakefulness and energy. No wonder you want to have sex all night! It also boosts serotonin, which makes you feel happy. PEA itself youthifies by increasing motivation, energy, emotions and the desire to connect with others. And even better, it curbs your appetite, boosts your metabolism and helps you lose weight. What's not to like?

Many researchers believe PEA can slow the ageing process and even increase lifespan. We know it makes us feel incredible. The PEA surge isn't the only way sex is good for us. Here are five more reasons:

- **Sex reduces stress**. The hormone oxytocin, which is released during sex, helps you relax and reduces anxiety. In a 2006 study at the University of Paisley, women who had sex at least once a week had lower blood pressure when subjected to stressful situations, such as public speaking, showing that women who have regular sex have better responses to stress than abstainers. Interestingly, intercourse was more effective against stress than any other type of sex.
- **Sex boosts your immunity**. Having sex once or twice a week has been linked with higher levels of an antibody called immunoglobulin A or IGA, which can protect you from infections. Non-stop sex, however, can reduce immunity – perhaps because you aren't getting enough sleep, which brings us to . . .
- **Sex helps you sleep**. Oxytocin promotes a desire to cuddle and connect, and it also promotes great sleep. As you know from our chapter on sleep,

getting enough sleep has been linked with a host of other good things, such as keeping you slim, while reducing your risk of disease.

- **Sex is a natural painkiller**. Oxytocin surges boost endorphins, and this is proven to dramatically reduce pain. That makes sex a natural solution to anything from period pains to a headache.

- **Sex makes you look young**. In a study at the Royal Edinburgh Hospital, women who had the most sex with their partners – four times a week, on average – were perceived by researchers to be seven to twelve years younger than their actual age. Why? It might be because sex boosts your levels of the sex hormones testosterone and oestrogen, which makes you feel sexier, and makes skin smoother, lips plumper and hair thicker.

- **Orgasms are good for the brain**. Ongoing research at Rutgers University in New Jersey shows that when women of any age have an orgasm, MRI scans show their entire brain lights up! The professor in charge of the research says, 'Orgasm brings all the nutrients and oxygenation to the brain. Mental exercises increase brain activity in localized regions. Orgasm activates the whole brain.' Plus it's more fun than a crossword.

You might not think this, given the impression the media gives that sex is just for the young, but there is plenty of evidence that sex can keep getting better as you get older. In 2000, US pollsters Yankelovich Partners interviewed women aged between fifty and sixty-five about sex. Overwhelmingly, they found that their sexual desire and interest in sex was undimmed, and had even increased since menopause. A staggering 82 per cent of women taking HRT said that their sex life had improved or stayed the same, compared to 68 per cent of women not taking HRT. And the women on HRT also had more sex than those who weren't.

So what makes a post-menopausal sex life so great? The women on HRT listed feeling comfortable with their partner, physical fitness, no fear of pregnancy and HRT as the top four reasons for loving their sex life. And 60 per cent of women on HRT said the treatment was more important to their sex life than sexy lingerie, though we think that can't hurt either.

Other reasons why women thought their sex life got better included better life balance, cited by 77 per cent, and kids being off their hands (61 per cent).

There are hormonal reasons why you can feel a surge of sexual power in mid-life, particularly in the peri-menopause, the time of hormonal shifts prior to the menopause. One is that you are more sensitive to that key sex hormone testosterone. All women produce testosterone, but when you are younger it's mopped up in our systems in the presence of high oestrogen. When your oestrogen levels fall, your testosterone becomes more potent, which can boost desire.

In addition to this, many women simply feel less shy and more confident as they get older, both about who they are and what they want in and out of bed. He's not hitting the spot? A twenty-something woman might lie back and just hope he gets there in the end, while a woman over forty is likely to give him a map.

Sex and Your Hormones

As we've seen, women taking hormone supplements have more desire. They also fantasize more, are more easily aroused, have more sex and enjoy it more. Oh, the joy! Oestrogen works on its own for many women, but oestrogen plus testosterone often works even better.

There is, however, another hormone-linked problem that many women discover as they age: vaginal dryness. While sex is more than intercourse, if your oestrogen levels are low then it can be harder to get wet, your vagina can actually get smaller and the skin can become thinner. This thinner skin produces less lubrication, making penetrative sex very unsexy, and even painful. Some women who think they have a dryness problem meet a new man and it disappears – it was just a lust problem. But if the problem isn't with desire, what options are there?

Some women find things get better if they eat a diet rich in plant oestrogens and take food supplements like soya or red clover. A simple, instant answer to dryness is to invest in a vaginal 'bio-adhesive' moisturizer – you'll find this at the chemist or you can buy it online – which makes sex sexily slippery. We know it doesn't sound very erotic, but this type of moisturizer is more than a lubricant; it contains ingredients that mean the cream can hold up to sixty times its weight of water, plus it sticks to the skin cells until they are naturally shed every two or three days. It can even reduce dryness in the long term. Dryness down there can also mean the pH of the vagina changes, so you become more prone to infections, but with a good moisturizer, the pH is kept naturally, healthily acidic.

Alternatively, see a specialist or your doctor about hormonal supplementation, either through HRT, bio-identical hormones or, if you are worried about adding hormones to your entire system (more about that later), you can be prescribed an oestrogen gel, cream or pessary that you apply directly to the vagina, which can really help.

But that's not all. We'd like to tell you about some very interesting, very new developments in medicine which focus on the specific changes that affect our bodies and our sex lives. Some of these are controversial, not because they don't work but, we think, because some people are pretty horrified that women who are mothers, or are older, still care about their sex lives. One treatment is a new type of filler that contains hyaluronic acid, a natural, water-attracting component of young skin, which can be injected by a gynaecologist into the vaginal wall to plump and moisturize it. Another is vaginal laser rejuvenation. Lasers down there may sound scary, but because the actual vaginal walls have no pain receptors, this treatment doesn't hurt. (Honest! In the course of our research, we've seen it done and talked to women who have had it.) It takes ten minutes, and, just like laser treatment for the face, boosts

Nope!

collagen and elastin, making the vaginal walls thicker, healthier and more moist, for up to two years – it may last longer, but as this is a new treatment doctors aren't sure how long the effects are sustained. Both the injection and the laser treatment tighten the vagina for more sensation during intercourse and should help reduce recurrent infections due to dryness and thinning.

The laser treatment also helps remodel the entire area, including the pelvic floor. Studies show that this type of treatment can dramatically reduce stress incontinence – the type that happens when you laugh, run, or dance. Some doctors estimate that between a third and two thirds of women suffer from some degree of stress incontinence as they get older or after childbirth. Stress incontinence can start to restrict what you do, make you self-conscious and feel less sexy. Pelvic floor exercises – explained further in this chapter so keep reading – can and do help most women (if they do them religiously), but for women who find that impossible, or find they don't work, these treatments could be the answer. Now, these treatments are new, and studies are ongoing, no we can't really recommend them yet, but they are certainly ones to keep an eye on for the future.

Can Supplements Spice Up Your Sex Life?

The menopause is a massive readjustment of body chemistry arising from dramatic changes in hormone levels during just a few years, but as we've seen, it doesn't have to harm your sex life. Obviously, how much you want and enjoy sex depends on lots of factors. Your relationship is obviously a key one. If you don't love, respect or fancy your partner, then you aren't likely to be having a sizzling sex life together. Stress, illness, exhaustion and certain medications can also take their toll, but it is clear that hormonal changes also play a big part, and there is evidence that certain supplements may be able to help.

DHEA

Remember DHEA, that hormone whose decline begins, rather steeply, in our twenties and keeps on dropping? The levels are down to about 50 per cent of their peak value when we are in our forties, and less than 20 per cent when we are in our seventies. DHEA is a precursor to the male sex hormone androstenedione, which in turn is a precursor to both testosterone and oestrogen.

It is known that many, but not all, users of DHEA – particularly women – notice an increase in libido when they take the supplement. This may be due to a significant increase in testosterone, which has a pro-sexual effect. The effect is more obvious in older women, who have been reported to experience not only increased desire, but also increased sexual activity and satisfaction.

When given doses of 25–50 mg a day of DHEA (in tablet form) for six months, post-menopausal women saw their menopausal symptoms improve and their sex lives see a boost.

In the US, the hormone DHEA is sold as a food

for future!

supplement, but it can only be obtained on private pre-scription in the UK.

L-arginine

This amino acid is converted in the body into a chemical called nitric oxide. Nitric oxide causes blood vessels to open wider for improved blood flow. L-arginine also stimulates the release of growth hormone, insulin and other sub-stances in the body. Better blood flow can make the clitoris and vagina more sensitive and responsive to sexual stimula-tion, so could increase your chances of reaching the big O.

It's been found that post-menopausal women who take a supplement including L-arginine experience heightened sexual response. When combined with L-lysine, L-arginine may also help reduce stress and anxiety, and cut the stress hormone cortisol. As our libidos are badly affected by stress and cortisol, this may also help boost libido. Foods rich in L-arginine include poultry, meats, fish, beans (espe-cially soya), grains, nuts and seeds.

You can find L-arginine supplements sold over the counter. It's an ingredient in the supplement YOUTH, developed by Dr Daniel Sister, where it's paired with L-lysine.

Sexercise?

Exercise is proven to help women like their bodies more because it helps you focus on what your body can do, rather than just what it looks like. So that's another reason to hit the gym or, even better, the yoga studio, as yoga's been proven to boost body image and reduce stress levels, which are known to reduce desire.

Exercise also increases blood flow – everywhere! – which is absolutely vital to arousal, as well as having a powerful hormonal effect. If you want to feel sexier, grab your weights and do some bicep curls. Why? Not only will you love your arms more, but weight training boosts levels of testosterone, a hormone that we know makes women feel sexier and improves blood flow to the areas that count.

Don't worry, weightlifting is not going to give you a burly build or a beard. The testosterone that's released is at healthy, natural levels. Too tired to exercise and too tired for sex? Exercise – as long as you don't overdo it – can boost your energy levels. If your tiredness is chronic, get more sleep, or if sleep's the only thing you're getting plenty of in bed, read on . . .

Love Yourself

We live in a world where we are constantly told that only women who look like Victoria's Secret models are sexy and sexual. Some younger people even think older women should retire from the sexual arena altogether. If you take these messages on board, it can affect your confidence and sense of attractiveness. This is why the key to a fantastic sex life as we get older is a good body image.

If you love your body, you are more able to let someone else love it, too. How can you love your body more? First of all, make a conscious decision to hold your head up high, refuse to apologize for your age and reject the idea of the 'perfect body' being the only one that deserves sexual pleasure.

There's no such thing as a perfect body – unless you actually are a Victoria's Secret model and, frankly, even they probably have bits of themselves they aren't crazy about – so *feeling* sexy is better than *looking* sexy. And you can feel sexier by building sensuality into your day and priming all the sensitive nerves in the skin of your whole body. Upgrade your shower gel to a scented oil, body brush to increase blood flow, wear underwear that makes you feel foxy, and clothes that are soft and feel good on your skin.

Spend time doing things you love, and allow yourself me-time, to relax, to de-stress and to let go of tension, which makes everyone feel less sexy. To eroticize your brain, read erotic books, see films with sexy characters and simply think about sex more. Studies show that erotic literature makes women feel sexier, and reading a self-help book about improving your sex life can have an even more powerful effect on your libido, which can translate into having more sex. If you still feel shy about your body in bed, you don't even have to get naked – beautiful underwear has an amazing effect on men.

A quick word here: we know that not all of you will have a partner, but you still deserve a great sex life. An orgasm is an orgasm, however you get there. That may be with someone else or it may be on your own. Your fingers, or a vibrator, can produce seriously satisfying orgasms, and if you want the cuddle fix that sex provides, remember that you get the same gorgeous oxytocin boost from any kind of touch. So get hugs from your friends and family, and book regular massages for your oxytocin fix, then come home and close the deal!

More is More

Perhaps the quickest way to feel sexier is simply to have more sex. As we've already explained, orgasm boosts the hormone oxytocin, which makes you want to get physically close, and creates a total dopamine brainstorm, so you'll want more orgasms.

It also boosts your levels of the hormone testosterone. Women have testosterone, too, and it has a powerful effect on our libido. Studies also show that the more you orgasm, the higher your testosterone levels are, and the higher they are, the more and more powerful orgasms you have. Plus women who boost their testosterone with sex report feeling much sexier the next day. Of course, if you feel sexy, you want more sex, and if sex makes you feel sexier . . . well, you get the picture.

A wise woman we know always advises her single girlfriends to give themselves an orgasm before they go out to a place where they might meet Mr Right. 'A woman who's just had an orgasm exudes sexuality and men love it,' she insists. And now we know she's right, scientifically.

Exercise also boosts PEA and testosterone, so a workout in the gym followed by a passionate encounter or a solo session can be the perfect combination to increase wellbeing and body confidence.

Dopamine is associated with excitement, so taking risks and doing new things will increase dopamine levels in the brain, while the same old, same old will reduce them. Playing games in bed, going on a rollercoaster together, having sex outdoors or just checking into a hotel can get levels up. To be honest, we can't think of a more powerful aphrodisiac than having sex in a bed that we haven't had to make ourselves.

Being bored, tired and resentful are sure ways to find your libido hits rock bottom. Make sure you get time with your man to have fun, and time for yourself. Eat and sleep well to raise your energy levels. Chronic dieting can have a devastating impact on your energy levels, metabolism and body image.

Also, your body needs some healthy fat to make your vital sex hormones. Of course, a great relationship makes the biggest difference. Studies show that, particularly after the menopause, women are more sexual with partners they feel truly loved by and safe with, and report much higher levels of desire if their man is romantic. Why not tell him that, and watch those flowers and chocolates roll in?

Why Don't I Want Sex?

If your libido has disappeared and these suggestions don't help, it's worth thinking about a medical reason for your flatlining sex drive. Here are some pretty common ones:

- **Hypothyroidism.** You've read how common it is to have a malfunctioning thyroid gland as you get older. Well, your thyroid hormones drive almost every function of your body, including your sex drive. Other symptoms are tiredness, weight gain and hair loss. Ask your doctor for a blood test.

- **Anaemia.** Low iron can nix your naughty thoughts, and you'll be too exhausted to contemplate a romp. If you don't eat red meat or take iron supplements, and especially if you still have periods, you may have low iron. If you are pale, tired and get short of breath, suspect anaemia. Again, a blood test can diagnose, and supplements and diet can treat.

- **Depression.** Loss of desire is a very common part of depression. If you have stopped feeling passion for anything in your life, including sex, see your doctor.

- **Medication.** The great irony about depression and lack of libido is that many anti-depressants can kill your sex drive stone dead. It's a well-known side effect. If this applies to you, talk to your doctor about a change of medication.

- **You're in an unhappy relationship**. OK, this isn't a medical reason. In fact, it's normal and healthy to lack desire if you are bored by, or don't like, love or respect, your partner. Couples counselling or specialist sex therapy may help reignite the flame if your relationship has just become stale or you aren't communicating. But if your relationship is emotionally dead, and particularly if it's physically abusive, you will always be happier, in and out of bed, as a single woman.

What If He Doesn't Want Sex?

This is a problem that's rarely talked about, but quite common. Men also suffer from stress, depression, body worries, hormone changes and medical conditions that can harm both sexual desire and physical arousal.

Men can be very ashamed of this and not want to seek help or even discuss it. If you want sex and he doesn't, then it might be time for a supportive, kind talk about how much you desire him, and how much you miss your sex life.

Try to get him to talk about why your sex life has flagged. If it's a physical problem with erection, then you can either decide to have sex other ways, or he can seek help via a doctor. Conditions like diabetes can damage blood flow, for example, while viagra can be successful in giving men their erection back.

Low testosterone can cause libidos and energy to flag. A GP or specialist hormone doctor can organize blood tests and carefully monitor testosterone replacement that can safely raise his hormone levels.

Encourage your man to have a healthy lifestyle. Too much alcohol and junk food can take away desire and performance, whereas exercise can boost blood flow and testosterone levels, especially if he hits the weights room. In addition to this, a better body can make him more confident in bed, just like us. Try to keep the intimacy in your relationship going even if you don't have sex. It's harder to get back to being passionate if your relationship has lost its romance, too.

Kiss It Better

Kissing is the ultimate aphrodisiac. It has the capacity to bridge conflicts and differences between people, to bring people closer and make both the kisser and the kissee feel better.

In a 2009 study at Rutgers University in the US (those Americans study so many things) people who kissed for fifteen minutes (you are allowed to come up for air) while listening to music experienced higher levels of oxytocin – the hormone that encourages you to bond – and lower levels of the stress hormone cortisol. The longer their relationship, the more the couples benefited hormonally.

Big, passionate kisses can even help you lose weight, as kissing increases your metabolic rate, therefore helping you burn calories. Kissing has also been proven to increase adrenaline, making your heart work faster and increasing blood flow. The results are lower blood pressure, lower cholesterol and better cardiovascular activity.

We strongly advise you to get out there and find that certain loved one, or 'in lust' one, to start kissing.

Fire Down Below

When it comes to fitness, Kegels count, too. These pelvic-floor-strengthening exercises can have big rewards when it comes to sexual satisfaction. Kegels consist of contracting and relaxing the muscles in your pelvic floor. Get them all toned up, and you will have more sexual pleasure and stronger orgasms, as well as keeping your bladder and sexual organs functioning in a healthy, youthful way.

So how do you do a Kegel?

- First imagine the muscles that control the start and stop of urine.
- If you don't know what we're talking about, try stopping in mid-flow next time you are on the loo, but only once or twice, as it's not good for you!
- Once you've found them, pull those muscles in and up.
- Hold for about five seconds, relax and then repeat.
- Ideally, repeat for at least five minutes every day.

Psst! You can do these anywhere – at home, in the office, on the train, even right now – and no one will know but you!

Take Control!

- Sex is great for your health and wellbeing, and practised regularly it can make you look up to twelve years younger.
- Exercise, especially weight training, boosts levels of your sexy hormones.
- Look out for emotional, psychological and physical reasons why your, or his, libido might be flagging.
- Think about hormone replacement for a sexier, happier you.
- The more you have, the more you want, so just do it.

'Sex is a part of nature. I go along with nature.'
Marilyn Monroe

9. Take Control: Exercise

How Exercise Can Boost Your Youth
Hormones and Reverse Ageing
Good News: You May Need to Sweat
Less than You Think

For some of you, the mere idea of exercise will make you want to put this book down and go back to bed. Sadistic PE teachers, a horror of Lycra and a belief that there's no point exercising if it doesn't hurt like hell can all put you off getting moving. But come on, you know us better than that by now. We aren't fanatics. We don't want you to do anything you hate. Also, we are as busy as you are. But the truth is, once we've explained just how important exercise is to your happy, healthy, young-at-any-age future, we know you will be inspired.

Personally, we have found that as we get older, we've become less obsessed with exercise as a way to look skinny and more interested in how it holds back and even reverses the ageing process. We don't want to be 'doddery' or 'frail' just because we're older. We want to be strong, vital, able to travel, run, stretch, climb stairs, hike, dance and generally live our lives with enthusiasm for as long as possible.

Leah's mother, who is at an age when plenty of women are thinking about stair lifts, is a role model for the value of exercise in transforming a woman's experience of the second phase of her life. She has exercised all her life, and even now takes regular professional ballet classes. This isn't just because it's her job. It's because she loves to move, and hates the way her body feels if she's not moving. The result? She is still a Pilates teacher and professional dancer, regularly appearing on stage at the Royal Opera House and Glyndebourne with people up to fifty years younger than she is, and yet she is just as vital as them.

Susie has taught Pilates for years, and remains strong and supple, with energy levels that wear out staff half her age. The truth is, if you want to live well and for longer, you just have to move your body. It doesn't matter if you don't lose an ounce, because exercise can transform your health whatever size you are.

And our really good news? It's never too late to start exercising, and you can get fit and change your hormones doing much less than you think.

Why You Need to Exercise

Exercise can add an average of seven years to your life expectancy, improves your health, your hormonal profile, reduces stress and even protects your telomeres from shortening, making you younger right down to your cellular level. It makes you look and feel sexier, and it can give you thicker, brighter skin and stronger bones.

Osteoporosis is a terrifying disease. Crumbling bones cause pain, make you shrink and can even leave you disabled. But a study at the University of Arizona proved that strength training and weight-bearing exercises can increase your bone mineral density even after the menopause and without hormone therapy.

Exercise also makes your skin heal faster. Have you started noticing that little cuts and wounds take longer to heal than when you were young? Regular exercise can speed healing by up to 25 per cent.

Another advantage: exercise protects your muscles. We start losing muscle from around the age of forty-five, at a rate of 1 per cent a year, but specifically weight or resistance training can actually reverse this process. In addition to this, moderate exercise causes muscles to suck up glucose in the blood at twenty times the normal rate, keeping our blood sugar at safe, healthy levels and preventing diabetes.

Exercise can also turn on fullness hormones. We assume exercise will make us hungry, but a 2013 study from the Japanese Morinomiya University of Medical Science found levels of a gut hormone called glucagon-like peptide (GLP-1) rose in middle-aged Japanese women after a bout of exercise. GLP-1 is important for making us feel full, and high levels seem to cause weight loss.

It also makes you feel sexier. Women who exercise report feeling more attractive and happier with their bodies, regardless of whether they lose weight or not.

Chairs are Deadly!

We love relaxing on the sofa as much as the next woman, but research shows that sitting down is a health time bomb.

We simply aren't designed to sit about, especially in that relatively modern invention, the comfy chair. Evolution designed human beings to be upright, running, walking or squatting to cook and care for children and, when we get tired doing those things, lying down sleeping.

If we are awake and not moving, it's unnatural, and electrical activity in our muscles drops – 'The muscles go as silent as those of a dead animal,' according to one researcher – while your calorie-burning rate plunges to about one per minute, a third of what it would be if you simply got up and walked about.

Shockingly, even one day of inactivity makes our blood sugar spike up to 26 per cent more than it does on active days. Our risk of obesity also starts to rise, as enzymes responsible for vacuuming up fat out of the bloodstream plummet, making levels of good cholesterol fall.

In studies, compared with the least sedentary, those who spent the most time sitting down had a 112 per cent greater risk of diabetes, a 147 per cent rise in heart attacks and strokes and a 90 per cent higher risk of death from a heart attack.

The solution? Move more! Set an alarm for every twenty minutes you are working at a desk, and get up. At work, you could run up and down the stairs, walk to another floor to get a drink, or talk to someone instead of sending an email, and once the buzzer's gone off twice, walk around the block. Why not have meetings outdoors on the move, instead of over coffee and biscuits? It's so much better for your health, and it's much more likely to spark creativity, too.

It's Never Too Late to Start

If you haven't been a lifelong runner or aerobics fiend, and you've hit your forties, fifties or later, it's easy to feel that it's too late to start getting fit. But you'd be so wrong. Exercising at any age can transform your future. We are all living longer, but we're not necessarily living better. Chronic diseases such as diabetes and heart disease are soaring, but a study in *Archives of Internal Medicine* suggests that being, or becoming, fit in middle age, even if you haven't previously bothered with exercise, can have a dramatic effect on your future health. The study, which tracked men and women from the age of forty-nine until they were in their seventies or eighties, found that those who were the least fit at forty-nine were most likely to have one of eight serious conditions, such as diabetes, cancer, heart disease and Alzheimer's. And they got them earlier.

It also showed that fitter people in middle age live longer and, more importantly, stay healthier for more of their life, with the fittest tending to develop illnesses only in the last five years of their lives, instead of the last ten, fifteen or twenty. Sporty elderly people have a life expectancy that's almost four years higher than their less active peers', and are often faster than younger athletes.

How Exercise Makes You Smarter

Started forgetting where you put those keys? Study after study has proved that exercising is the most important way to keep your brain sharp and young and your memory working better as you get older.

Loss of oestrogen after the menopause can cause memory to decline, but tests on over-sixty-five-year-olds showed that regular walking actually increased the size of the hippocampus (the part of the brain that controls memory and other intellectual functions). In a 2012 Japanese study people aged between sixty-five and ninety-three were either given supervised exercises, involving aerobic, strength training and posture work, for ninety minutes once a week, or no exercise. At the end of twelve months, the group who had exercised had better memory and language skills.

A 2012 study at the University of British Columbia in Vancouver, Canada, looked at previously sedentary women between the ages of sixty and seventy with mild memory problems. They were asked to do either resistance training such as weightlifting, aerobic training such as walking, or balance and toning exercises, twice weekly for six months. Resistance training significantly improved attention, memory and other brain functions. Also, when the women's brains were scanned, three brain regions involved in memory showed increased activity. Aerobic training also improved their memories. The brains of exercisers were actually bigger, too. A more recent study has found that just six minutes of exercise – in the study they used an exercise bike – dramatically improved the memories of people over seventy.

Researchers believe that exercise is the best weapon we have in the war against the terrifying disease Alzheimer's. A 2003 University of California study of 6,000 women age sixty-five and older, over an eight-year period, found that women who were more physically active were less likely to see their mental function decline.

Physical activity seems to be more important than keeping the mind active with intellectual puzzles. A five-year study at Laval University in Sainte-Foy, Quebec, suggests that the protective effect of exercise on the brain is greater for women than men, and that while all exercise is protective, exercising vigorously three times a week could cut the risk of Alzheimer's in half. And if that isn't an incentive to pull on your trainers, frankly, we don't know what is.

One of the reasons exercise is so fantastic for the brain is that it stops the brain shrinking, which has a devastating effect on our sleep and memory. Exercise can even create new brain cells. It's long been known that the production of stem cells in the hippocampus area of the brain falls as we age, and that exercise can slow and even reverse that decline. Indeed, a few months of exercise can create new neurons. There is a vast body of evidence showing that exercise also reduces stress, anxiety and depression.

A 2012 study from the University of Edinburgh found that people over seventy who took regular exercise had less brain shrinkage over a three-year period than those who did little exercise. And the fit over-seventies taking regular exercise had more grey matter (the part of the brain with nerve cell bodies).

As we've said before, this doesn't have to be hard exercise. A 2011 study at the Beckman Institute at the University of Illinois of 120 older men and women who took up walking, found that after a year the walkers had a larger hippocampus in the brain and did better in tests of memory and thinking. Scans showed that they'd actually reversed the ageing process, making their hippocampus two years younger.

A 2011 study found that exercise triggers stem cells to become bone, not fat. The research, published by the *Journal of the Federation of American Societies for Experimental Biology*, found that under the influence of exercise, the stem cells became bone marrow cells, producing healthy blood that boosts the immune system.

In addition, exercise makes you shrug off stress. A 2013 study from researchers at Princeton University found that exercise 'reorganizes' the brain to reduce its response to stress and cut anxiety.

Less is More – The Amazing Exercise Paradox

OK, so exercise is essential. But pushing yourself too much could be harmful. Too much hard exercise may actually increase your cortisol levels, damage your heart, stop you losing weight and harm your health.

Be aware, though, we aren't talking about gentle jogging here, but serious training. For example, immediately after running a marathon, levels of an enzyme released when the heart is in distress soar by up to 50 per cent. This can signal that the overtaxed heart muscles are actually starting to tear, and in the end, this can leave the heart permanently damaged. When it comes to running, the optimum 'dose' of exercise appears to be about 10–15 miles a week, or a couple of miles a day.

While runners lived longer than non-exercisers, those who ran more than this did worse than the moderate exercisers. This perfect balance between being too sedentary and overdoing things is known as 'the Goldilocks zone' – not too lazy, not too frenetic, but just right! For your health, the ideal exercise prescription is from fifteen minutes to an hour a day, several days a week.

Even if you want to lose weight, less is more. A Danish study, as reported in the *Telegraph*, showed that people who worked out for thirty minutes a day lost more weight than those who exercised for an hour. Why? It seems too much exercise just makes you hungrier, so you eat more and cancel out any benefits of exercise on weight. The hour-a-day exercisers also appeared absolutely shattered, so when they weren't working out, they were glued to the sofa. The thirty-minutes-a-day exercisers, on the other hand, were far more lively once they started exercising, choosing the stairs over the lift and generally moving about more during the day. Another reason why excess exercise can stop you losing weight is that it causes a release of the stress hormone cortisol, which boosts fat storage.

Also, if you do a medium- to high-intensity workout for forty-five minutes or more, your body starts eating into your muscle tissue as a fuel source. This will cause you to lose the very active muscle tissue that helps you lose fat in the first place. One pound of muscle can burn 50–100 calories a day when you're doing nothing, so it's useful to build it up slowly.

Even your mental health depends on not overdoing exercise. In a study published in the journal *Prevention*, those who exercised for more than an hour a day had worse mental health than those who exercised for between 2.5 and 7.5 hours a week. This might be because they had body-dissatisfaction problems, were obsessive or simply because they didn't have enough time left over for fun, family and friends, and, as we know, fun and laughter are very good for your health.

The Science of Fast Fitness

OK, we now know you can exercise too much, but imagine fitting an entire week's workout into less time than it takes to get changed into your gym kit. Now imagine that this workout has more benefits than slogging it out in an hour-long exercise class.

Luckily, this type of fast, effective exercise isn't a fantasy. The latest buzzword in fitness is High Intensity Training, or HIT. HIT can yield many of the health and fitness benefits you would expect from four to five hours' training, but in just three to ten minutes per week. Not only that, but this short and not-very-sweet regime keeps telomeres shorter and generally makes your body younger. HIT means exercising as hard as you can for twenty to thirty seconds, resting for a couple of minutes and then repeating this between two and ten times. This type of exercise boosts your insulin function, is great for building muscle and increases your body's production of human growth hormone (HGH), which is associated with lower body fat, more lean muscles, higher energy and an enhanced immune system.

When it comes to controlling your weight, HIT also wins, because unlike lengthy workout sessions that can leave you hungry and under the mistaken impression you can afford to eat what you want, short bursts of intense activity don't affect your appetite as dramatically.

HIT raises metabolism for much longer after exercise than moderate intensity programmes (six to eight hours compared to one to two hours), which means more fat is burned, and if you are busy, it's brilliant as it takes up far less of your day. Intense exercise is also a powerful calorie burner. Researchers at Colorado State University say that 2.5 minutes of HIT exercise done in thirty-second bursts can burn up to 200 calories.

A homemade HIT session might involve jogging gently for a couple of minutes before sprinting or running up the stairs as fast as you can for thirty seconds, jogging or walking for a minute, then sprinting or stair climbing; repeating the whole thing three to five times, and doing this three times a week.

So why does HIT work so well? It seems rapid bursts of muscle movement appear to flood the blood with hormones called catecholamines. These break down stored fat in the body and burn it up as energy. What's more, drinking green tea after exercise appears to keep the levels of those fabulous fat-burning catecholamines high – so you continue burning fat even after you stop exercising.

To get the best from HIT, don't eat for an hour before or after your workout to avoid an insulin surge, which may prevent the release of fat-burning hormones. There are some disadvantages to HIT, mainly that the exercise has to be super-intense to work. You absolutely have to run, jump or cycle to the point where you think your heart might burst, so it's not good if you are very overweight, unfit, have injuries, or if you simply hate it. Always check with your doctor before starting any new exercise programme.

If pushing yourself to your limit gives you a buzz, HIT is perfect for you. If you find it unpleasant or stressful, you'll just pour out stress hormones like cortisol and you'd be better off, healthwise and hormonally, opting for gentler exercise.

Exercise and Fat Around the Middle

We know that in mid-life we tend to gain fat around the waist. Yes, the dreaded middle-aged spread. And we know that the fat we gain here can be particularly dangerous to our health, wrapping around our internal organs and pouring out inflammatory chemicals that lead to insulin resistance. This makes it easier to gain weight and harder to lose it: a vicious circle that can lead to diabetes. The cure? Exercise.

Numerous studies show that even moderate exercise, the equivalent of a gentle jog or fast walk, dramatically reduces belly fat. And it works. Those who do simple aerobic exercise, just enough to get you slightly out of breath, for at least thirty minutes three times a week can reduce their visceral or internal fat levels by between 25 and 60 per cent. Many of these studies showed that exercisers lost all their fat from the inside, including fat actually in the liver.

Why Exercise Isn't Enough

As we age we not only have to change what we eat but also how we move, stand, breathe and exercise. Exercise has to be fun or you won't stick to it, so find something you enjoy doing, from tennis to golf, hiking, cycling, gym, Pilates, yoga, swimming. Basically, anything that gets you moving is good, and the best part is that you can incorporate it into your daily life. But remember what we said about those deadly chairs? If you spend most of your life sitting, you need to think beyond exercise and focus on simply moving your body. Ensure you get up from your desk at least once every hour, have meetings as you walk, stroll to your destination instead of grabbing a cab, take the stairs not the lift, cycle to work, go pull out some weeds, meet a friend at a gallery not a restaurant, and walk to the shops instead of taking the car. We've seen people's health transformed by getting a dog!

So, even if you hate the gym or running, this sort of brisk but easy activity can alter your biology, improve your blood pressure, cholesterol and hormone balance and keep your weight steady.

Stretch Yourself Young

Young bodies are supple, flexible bodies. Being stiff and unable to reach or bend easily can make anyone appear absolutely ancient. Susie and Leah 'stretch every morning when we wake up and again after exercise. Or just when we feel the need.' 'I spend so much time hunched over a desk,' says Leah, 'so I do stretches that push my back in the opposite direction. Nothing makes you look older or feel worse than a stoop.'

Both yoga and Pilates are excellent for flexibility. It's well worth finding a great personal trainer, yoga or Pilates instructor and taking a few lessons in stretching. If you have a problem, such as a bad back, they can also give you specialist exercises and stretches to help.

It's invigorating, both physically and mentally, and not only does it enhance your exercise performance, it can decrease injury and minimize muscle soreness, too. Stretching increases the length of our muscles, which gives us that long lean look, and it also reduces muscle tension and increases our normal range of movement. By increasing your range of movement you are increasing the distance your limbs can move before damage to the muscles and tendons occurs.

Remember, like anything else new, stretching correctly is vital. Stretch only to the point of tension, never to the point of pain, and always warm up prior to stretching. Warm muscles are like plasticine, they stretch better than cold ones. So don't stretch before your run, but afterwards.

Beautiful Bones

Your bone structure is more than how great your cheekbones look. Strong bones are vital as we get older, and exercise protects bone density. A 2012 study at Glasgow Caledonian University found that even in women with osteoporosis, gentle weight training can slow bone degeneration. All types of exercise from aerobics to t'ai chi helped make bones stronger. As lower oestrogen levels cause bone loss, it's yet another reason to consider hormone supplements, especially if you are thin, obese, have taken steroid medication or smoke, all of which increase your risk of osteoporosis.

If you have a family history of osteoporosis – a granny with a bent spine or a mother with fractures – then you should ask your doctor for bone-density checks from your fifties or even earlier. Otherwise, start getting them in your sixties. There are a variety of drugs, as well as hormones, that can help, but prevention is of the essence as nothing can turn weak bones back into strong ones.

Your Weekly Exercise Prescription

For ultimate health and anti-ageing benefits this is the perfect balance of cardio, strength and balance training.

- Lots of everyday movement.
- Forty-five minutes of HIT or between 2.5 and 7.5 hours of moderate aerobic exercise for heart and lung health.
- Try to include lifting weights at least once a week, as it can boost your testosterone to healthy levels, which is good for sex drive and energy, builds muscle to burn calories and improves strength, and helps to improve your balance and tones your body.

- Take up yoga, t'ai chi, ballet or Pilates for balance, mental health and to reduce stress and cortisol.
- Work out outdoors when you can, ideally in the morning, to set your melatonin-led sleep/wake cycle and improve your mood.

The Hormone Power of Posture

Great posture is exercise. By standing tall with your shoulders back you instantly look younger and slimmer. Holding in your stomach and bottom as you stand, sit and walk keeps muscles firm and protects your back.

Fascinating research has found that you can change your hormonal balance simply by changing the way you sit and stand. Researcher Amy Cuddy, a psychologist at the Harvard Business School, found that if women adopted stereotypically male 'power postures', such as standing behind a desk, leaning forward with their hands resting on the table, their testosterone levels increased and levels of the stress hormone cortisol fell.

The women reported feeling more confident and powerful and researchers found they were more willing to take risks. But if they were asked to adopt meek postures, such as sitting with legs and arms folded, the reverse happened. This had nothing to do with being seen to be powerful, as the study participants were alone, but about their own self-perception. It seems that postures that involve taking up more space in the world give the best results. So standing tall is important. Yoga poses that take up space, such as the Warrior Pose and the Sun Salute, are likely to give a similar hormonal boost.

Three Power Postures to Try

- When sitting on a chair with arms, place your hands on the armrests, opening up your chest. Sit upright, not leaning forward.
- Stand tall, with feet slightly apart, back straight and head aligned with your spine.
- Let your hands relax, with open fingers rather than a tense clenched fist. Don't clutch your hands together or hold your hands to your chest. Make bold gestures when you speak.

How Fish Oils Can Double the Benefit of Exercise

We know we keep talking about oily fish, but here's another reason to eat salmon or mackerel three times a week: it can make your exercise regime twice – yes twice! – as effective.

After your mid-thirties, it's harder to build muscle during exercise. But in a 2012 study at Aberdeen University, older women who took fish oil as well as a twice-weekly thirty-minute workout improved their muscle strength by 20 per cent, compared to just 11 per cent in those who didn't take supplements. After twelve weeks, the exercisers who took fish oils also made bigger improvements to their balance, walking speed and the alacrity with which they were able to spring from their chairs.

You know what we really love about this study? The women, all of whom were in their sixties, improved their fitness this much simply by exercising for one hour a week. And let's face it, we can all do that.

Take Control!

- Make a commitment to move more. You don't just need exercise, you need to be more active in your daily life.
- If you work at a desk, set a timer and move every twenty minutes. Take a walk and stretch every forty minutes.
- Stand tall. Posture makes you stronger, slimmer and improves your hormone balance.
- Mix up your exercise. Try to incorporate aerobic exercise, which can be brisk walking or jogging, weight training and some kind of stress-relieving posture-based exercise, such as yoga or Pilates, into your week, as well as stretching.
- If you have a physical weakness, such as a bad back or weak ankles, see a physiotherapist or a qualified personal trainer who can give you specialist exercises to help.

'Old age is no place for sissies.'
Bette Davis

10. Take Control: Inflammation

Hey, we've gone on about it long enough by now, so we are sure you totally get that ageing is not a straightforward matter of how many candles are on your birthday cake; nor is it a disease. Of course, hormone changes have a lot to do with how you look and feel as the years go by, but some scientists claim that much of what you think of as ageing is actually 'inflamm-ageing'. You may not have heard of it, but it's a big buzzword in modern ageing science.

Inflammation may even be the source of many chronic conditions that you tend to think of as diseases of ageing. These include diabetes, Alzheimer's, arthritis and rheumatism, obesity, heart disease and even, yup, wrinkles. Guess what? Inflammation is linked to our hormones, particularly oestrogen, so women are more likely to fall victim to many inflammatory conditions.

What Is Inflamm-Ageing?

You know how when you get stung by a wasp, your skin becomes red and swollen? That's inflammation. Your body produces chemicals that make blood flow to the damaged area and change the way your cells work. If this didn't happen, injuries would never heal.

You can take drugs called 'anti-inflammatories' to calm pain and swelling, but as you get older and your immune system becomes less effective, instead of just appearing when we have an injury, inflammation starts to stick around all the time.

How can you tell? You might get achy muscles, swollen joints, stomach problems, or skin redness. All of these are inflammatory conditions. When inflammation isn't just a response to an injury and never totally goes away, the condition is called chronic or low-grade inflammation. Your body keeps on producing those inflammatory chemicals, including cytokines, which tell cells to die, and free radicals, which damage cells. This leads to damage throughout your entire body, including your stomach, blood vessels, skin and organs.

Chronic inflammation is linked to a host of immune disorders, such as rheumatoid arthritis, fibromyalgia, high blood pressure, lupus, plus heart disease, depression and obesity. It sounds scary, but there is actually some good news. Inflammation is treatable, and this means you can take control of a key component of the ageing process. You can make yourself younger, inside and out.

What Makes Inflammation Worse?

Guess what? It's those old enemies rearing their ugly heads again. Causes of chronic inflammation include lack of exercise, smoking, stress, too much alcohol, bad diet and lack of sleep. Causes of skin inflammation include pollution, UV light and harsh skincare. Food is a leading cause of internal inflammation, and here are the worst culprits:

Trans Fats

These are highly toxic and highly inflammatory. These partially hydrogenated vegetable oils are found in some processed foods, such as biscuits, and are linked to heart disease. Many studies show a mere 2 per cent increase in trans-fat consumption increases a woman's risk of heart disease by 93 per cent. How shocking is that?

Sugar

Inflammation starts to rise if you eat as little as a spoonful of sugar a day. Insulin spikes caused by sugar or refined, white carbs cause inflammation and ageing, and reduce the amount of antioxidants in your blood. Sugar is also ageing for our skin, as it triggers a process in the body called glycation. Sugar molecules bind to your springy and bouncy collagen and elastin fibres, which are the building blocks of skin, making them stiff and brittle so they break. As a result, skin starts to sag and wrinkle.

The glycation process creates harmful new molecules called advanced glycation end products (AGEs). The body treats these as invaders and responds by causing further inflammation and damage to your collagen and elastin. Can you imagine a more ageing food than a deep-fried dough-nut? Which brings us to . . . barbecued and fried food. Steak and chips? Gorgeous! But also, tragically, ageing. Cooking food at very high temperatures creates AGEs, as does any food that's browned, even pastry or a baked potato.

Cut down on browned food, especially if it's high GI and causes blood sugar spikes. Cook at lower temperatures and eat more steamed and raw food. But don't worry, we aren't saying you should never eat chips or a baked potato again! Just think of food like this as an occasional treat, not a regular staple.

Salt

Chips with lots of salt? Yes, delicious, but studies show that eating too much salt is linked to inflammation. We all need some salt, but avoid salty processed meats and ready meals (you know that, right?) and if you are a saltaholic, like Leah, try to get used to shaking less on your food. Use herbs and pepper instead. And to help persuade you: pepper boosts metabolism and aids digestion.

How to Fight Inflammation – Foods that Heal

A key weapon against inflammation is antioxidants. These powerful, vital chemical compounds are found in natural, healthy foods, particularly vegetables and fruit, and they naturally reduce inflammation by deactivating free radicals. Natural plant foods also contain inflammation-lowering doses of fibre and the mineral magnesium. You should aim to eat five to nine portions of vegetables and fruit a day. Use colour as your guide to mix them up for maximum effect.

Omega-3 Fatty Acids

Both from oily fish and in supplement form, these turn down your inflammatory response. Aim for two 3–4 oz servings of oily fish such as salmon or fresh tuna a week. In other studies, eating nuts reduces inflammation. Polyunsaturated fatty acids, antioxidant vitamins, fibre, the amino acid L-arginine and the mineral magnesium are all potent anti-inflammatories, and nuts contain them all!

Get Spicy

Polyphenols are inflammation-dampening antioxidants, and spices such as turmeric, garlic and ginger are rich in them, as well as being delicious.

Virgin Olive Oil

It's becoming clear that virgin olive oil is powerfully anti-inflammatory and helps prevent disease. A recently discovered compound in olive oil is oleocanthal. This has similar anti-inflammatory and pain-relieving effects to ibuprofen and aspirin, but without their side effects. The darker and stronger the oil, the more anti-inflammatory it is. About 3.5 tablespoons of olive oil is equivalent to a 200 mg tablet of ibuprofen. That's a lot of calories, though, so think about using a couple of tablespoons of strong olive oil to replace other oils in salad dressings or on cooked vegetables, and use it as a spread on wholegrain bread. It's one of the key ingredients that make the Mediterranean diet so healthy.

Inflammation and Your Weight

Insulin resistance, as we've said, is caused when our bodies have been called on to pump out too much insulin for too long, and in the end the sheer quantity means our cells become 'resistant', or immune, to the hormone and stop responding to it.

Not realizing this, the pancreas pumps out even more until it collapses and stops functioning. The result? Diabetes. At the same time, you tend to become resistant to the fullness hormone leptin, so you eat more. And your poor old overstuffed fat cells start to pour out cytokines, or inflammatory chemicals. This may be a vicious circle, where a bad diet – refined carbs, sugar and trans fats – contributes to inflammation, potentially increasing insulin and leptin resistance.

The theory is that junk food upsets the vital balance of our digestive bacteria, causing the growth of internal gut bacteria, which cause inflammation. We are colonized by more bacteria than you can imagine. Too much information, perhaps, but half our – ahem – stool consists of live bacteria.

To fight inflammation, we need to get our gut bacteria back in balance. We'll talk about healthy foods and prebiotics, such as the plant fibres found in bananas, garlic, onions and asparagus, in Chapter 11. These are the perfect foods to feed the inflammation-quelling bacteria we need.

Also, treating inflammation is pretty much bound to have an effect on your weight. For example, we know junk food and stress make you fatter, as well as creating inflammation, but exercise is anti-inflammatory, as is sleep, and both help keep you thinner.

Fitness and Inflammation

Study after study show that exercise reduces chronic inflammation, as measured by markers of inflammation in the blood, such as C-reactive protein.

Resistance training, aerobic exercise and moderate cardio programmes all reduce inflammation and improve health, even if you don't lose weight. However, don't overdo it. Overly vigorous exercise actually increases markers of acute inflammation.

The key to managing inflammation with exercise is to do enough, but not too much, and rest in between. Walking and yoga are proven to reduce stress and inflammation, both while you are doing them and afterwards too. This makes them super-anti-agers. Just don't forget your sunscreen if you're outdoors.

Try to Keep Your Weight Down

It's hard, we know, but fat cells, especially the ones you tend to gain in mid-life around your middle, pour out inflammatory compounds such as histamines and cytokines. You know the sore knees that obese people often suffer? Don't assume they're caused by wear and tear – inflammation is a more likely culprit. If you can't get your weight down, then take exercise and eat well, as you can be big, but still have low inflammation if you live healthily. And by cutting inflammation, you could find it easier to manage your weight, too.

Sleep Away Inflammation

Insomnia sends your production of inflammatory cytokines soaring. This is why people with conditions such as back pain and arthritis feel much worse after a bad night's sleep. Sleep also switches off cortisol, the stress hormone, which triggers inflammation. Poor sleep causes high blood pressure, too. You know the deal. Aim for seven to eight hours of good-quality shut-eye.

Stress and Inflammation

Here's a big reason to try to calm down. Stress causes inflammation, and so does depression, which can be caused by stress. New research published in *Proceedings of the National Academy of Sciences* shows that chronic stress makes the body lose the ability to control inflammation. The culprit? Cortisol – again. Cortisol suppresses the immune system, which should cool inflammation down. But if we make too much cortisol our immune cells become immune to the hormone and inflammation gets out of control.

Want to know something surprising? Do you think you catch the worst colds when you are stressed? Actually, the severity of the symptoms is not caused by the type of virus you've got, but by the inflammatory response of your body. So if you are already in a chronic state of inflammation, you won't get more colds than anyone else, but your cold symptoms will be much worse.

Aspirin and Inflammation?
Should You Be Taking a Daily Dose?

Aspirin (acetylsalicylic acid) is naturally derived from willow bark and is an anti-inflammatory drug first used as a painkiller more than a century ago. It's been dubbed 'the ultimate anti-inflammatory', and studies have found that it can dramatically cut your risk of cancer, stroke, Parkinson's disease, heart disease and other conditions. It also lowers blood pressure, even in pregnancy.

Excitingly, in 2013, researchers at Oxford University found that taking low doses of aspirin for five years reduces the risk of death from cancer by a staggering 37 per cent overall. It reduces the risk of cancer of the colon (by up to 70 per cent), and oesophagus and breast cancer, among others. Encouragingly, aspirin also inhibits the growth of ovarian tumours by as much as 68 per cent. And what's more, if you do develop cancer and you regularly take aspirin, you may halve the risk of that cancer spreading to other parts of your body.

Overall, taking a daily aspirin for five or six years over a twenty-year period. seems to prevent around one in thirty deaths from cancer. Just a small, 75-mg daily dose of aspirin, taken over ten years or so, may reduce the risk of around half of cancers forming.

Even tiny doses seem to have a powerful effect. People who take aspirin for just one day a month – that's right, one dose a month – reduce their risk of heart disease by 35 per cent, compared to people who almost never use it. It works by thinning the blood, so it doesn't clot and block arteries. The same dose seems to reduce the risk of pancreatic cancer by 26 per cent, and two aspirin a week reduces the risk of Parkinson's disease in women by 40 per cent.

On the downside, though, aspirin can harm the lining of your stomach, causing stomach ulcers and internal bleeding, and trigger asthma attacks; in addition to this, people who take aspirin for a year or more are five times as likely to develop Crohn's disease. There is also some inconclusive research linking aspirin with a greater risk of pancreatic cancer in women, so you should always check with your doctor before taking any medication, including aspirin.

major downside.

If you're wondering, 'Should I take it?' the official advice is not to if you don't have a specific risk factor, such as a high risk of heart disease or cancer. Many people still do, though, Susie included, who, under medical advice, decided the benefits were too great to pass up. She takes 75 mg of aspirin daily, the same amount as is used in cancer prevention research. Peter Rothwell, who led the Oxford University research, suggests healthy people might start taking aspirin in their mid-forties, as the risk of dying from cancer rises from your fifties onwards. He also takes 75 mg a day himself, but advises people to talk to their GP before doing the same.

Take Control!

- Get more antioxidants in the form of fruit and vegetables.
- Swap bad hydrogenated fats for olive oil, nuts and nut oils, avocado and coconut oil.
- Don't eat white! Cut out refined carbs and sugar. If you want to eat carbs, pick low-GI, unrefined carbs, such as beans and wholegrains, to smooth blood sugar spikes. Eat lean protein and get more oily fish.
- Feed your good bacteria and soothe inflammation with fibre (supplements of konjac root are a source of insoluble fibre) as well as lots of fruit and vegetables.
- Don't smoke.
- Protect your skin with sunscreen.
- Exercise – but not too much.
- Sleep well.
- Consider taking a small daily dose of aspirin – but talk to your GP first.
- Try not to worry!

'I'm not interested in age. People who tell me their age are silly. You're as old as you feel.'
   Elizabeth Arden

11. Take Control: Hormone Therapy

Leah and Susie have done a great deal of research on this particular subject. It's a controversial area and new evidence is constantly evolving, but the key things we believe are that everyone is an individual and every body is different.

How your changing hormones affect you is unique. Every decision you make about whether or not to take hormone therapy, which type you choose, or whether to use alternative methods to support your body through the changes, must be taken in partnership with your doctor. This chapter simply aims to empower you by giving you the knowledge and understanding you need to make an informed decision and demand the best care from your doctor.

Why Would You Consider Taking Hormones?

Levels of our natural hormones start to decline from our twenties onwards, so it's no wonder we start to notice things changing by the time we hit our forties and fifties. After the age of about forty, for many of us there is a marked decrease in hormone production, and with it may come a broad spectrum of age-related symptoms and a decline in our youthful vitality.

Typically symptoms of hormone deficiencies may include:

- Hot flushes
- Tiredness
- Lack of libido
- Weight gain
- Dry skin
- Wrinkles
- Thinning hair
- Loss of muscle tone
- Vaginal dryness
- Osteoporosis
- High cholesterol
- Rising risk of heart disease

Do We Age Because Our Hormone Production Slows Down, Or Does It Slow Down Because We Are Getting Older?

Whatever the answer is, many researchers believe that a lot of the signs of ageing, such as shrinking muscle mass and decreasing bone density, are related to this age-associated decline in hormone production. We understand that it looks all doom and gloom, but hey, nobody gets all of these symptoms and some women, like Susie, don't really get any.

However, even with a healthy diet and lifestyle, most women do get some menopausal symptoms that impact on their health and happiness, so it's no wonder that when hormone replacement was developed, many women embraced it as a way to restore their quality of life.

The Hormone Controversy

In 2002, a study emerged that terrified those women. The Women's Health Initiative Study depicted hormone replacement as a killer. It claimed that HRT raised the risk of breast cancer by 26 per cent, and that it also increased the risk of heart disease and strokes. Overnight, women threw away their hormones and decided instead to endure those hot flushes, vaginal dryness, weaker bones and all the rest. But it was worth it, right?

Well, despite the scare, some doctors continued to point out that if maintaining youthful levels of hormones through the menopause was so dangerous, how come younger women are so healthy, vigorous and well? And how come your disease risk only really ramps up as your hormone levels start to slide? To doctors like Dr Sister and many others, hormones have never been scary, horrible killers, but the elixir of life and youth. It's not taking hormones that's dangerous; it's taking the wrong hormones, at the wrong time or in the wrong dosage.

Sometimes the science is wrong, too. Now we know the consequences of all those doctors taking women off hormones without considering their individual circumstances. In fact, new evidence has revealed that many women have died, yes died, prematurely and quite unnecessarily because they didn't take hormones. How many? Prepare to be shocked.

In 2013, a study by researchers at Yale University published in the *American Journal of Public Health* found that over a ten-year span, beginning in 2002, a minimum of 18,601 and as many as 91,610 post-menopausal women aged between fifty and fifty-nine years old died prematurely – mostly of heart disease – because they avoided HRT. And that's in the US. Can you imagine the numbers if we included every other country in the world? We find this statistic horrific. To make matters worse, the study was limited to women who'd become menopausal after hysterectomies. At the start of the study they were aged between fifty and fifty-nine years old. None of them lived into their seventies. We call that dying far too young.

The Yale study is not alone in drawing attention to death rates in women not taking HRT. In 2012 a Danish study was published in the *British Medical Journal*. It looked at women aged between forty-five and fifty-eight who took hormones for ten years immediately after the menopause and found that they had far less chance of having heart disease or of dying of a heart attack than women who were not on HRT.

In fact, the risk was nearly cut in half, and what's more they got this benefit with absolutely no extra risk of developing cancer, including breast cancer, getting a deep-vein thrombosis or having a stroke! Most importantly, the study found that even sixteen years later, there was still no extra risk of cancer, strokes or blood clots. Using HRT halved the risk of heart disease and strokes, and cut the death rate by a staggering 43 per cent. This figure echoes a 2010 statement issued by The Endocrine

Society in the US, which stated that hormone therapy was associated with a 40 per cent reduction in mortality when taken by women aged under 60, and that there was no increase in cardiovascular disease.

During the study period women had an improved quality of life and reduced their risk of dementia and broken bones. Yes, doctors have learned a lot about the right doses and formulation of hormone replacement in those ten years, and it isn't medically advised for all women, but it is still possible that hormone phobia may have led to many fabulous women dying before their time, which we think is a tragedy.

But what about that previous study, which claimed hormone replacement doubled the risk of breast cancer? How could it be so wrong? There are several reasons. Firstly, there were problems with how the results were interpreted, but also, researchers wanted to look at the effects of hormones on heart disease. To do this, they deliberately recruited women who were most at risk of heart attacks: women in their sixties. These women had been post-menopausal for ten years, though, so the scenario was completely artificial. Women never normally start wanting to take hormones a decade *after* their menopause. These women were not on HRT and hadn't planned to be, and it is likely that many of them were already developing hormone-deficiency conditions. For example, they had ten years to build up plaque in their arteries. If they then started taking oral oestrogen, this would have caused the plaque to become unstable, potentially causing heart attacks. Studies show that synthetic progestins increase breast cancer, while bio-identical progesterone does not. Also, when it comes to our health, it's important to realize that three times as many women die of heart disease than of breast cancer.

Also, importantly, the women in the study were using conventional HRT. More specifically, a formulation of HRT called Prempro. Prempro is a combination of oestrogens called conjugated equine oestrogens that are derived from the urine of pregnant horses, plus a synthetic progestegen called progestin, instead of natural progesterone. These synthetic hormones are not the same as your natural hormones and may have different effects. Synthetic oral oestrogen is metabolized in the liver, where it increases the formation of clotting proteins. Transdermal oestrogen does not. And bio-identical oestrogen is safer still.

So what should have been done differently? As a hormone specialist and medical doctor, Dr Daniel Sister believes that for optimum health at menopause, you should never aim to jolt your body back out of menopause many years after your ovaries have shut up shop. Instead, the ideal is to keep your hormones at healthily youthful levels throughout the menopause transition, depending on your own personal profile. You will have noticed that not only were all the women on one type of HRT, but the hormones used weren't chemically the same as human ones. Dr Sister has long rejected this type of conventional hormone therapy that we refer to as HRT.

Not every woman should – or can – take hormones. For women who have no symptoms and feel great, why would they want to? But if you have had a premature menopause or have thinning bones, then hormone therapy is strongly advised. If you have menopausal symptoms, but have had certain cancers or hormone-induced blood clots in the past, then any decisions must be made very carefully indeed and in consultation with a specialist. We couldn't possibly advise you either way here.

You see, Dr Sister believes that every woman taking hormones needs a personal hormone prescription, one that looks at her own individual symptoms and hormone profile, and which addresses all her hormonal, medical and lifestyle issues.

This doesn't mean that you will need to take dozens of supplements, but he believes the one-size-fits-all approach to hormone supplementation belongs in the Dark Ages.

To Dr Sister, hormone replacement is an art. He doesn't say, 'Oh, the numbers on this test say you are normal, so go away.' Instead, he looks at your body and at your symptoms, and works to restore your youthful health and function. And he can adjust the dosage as your body ages and changes. 'Your hormones work together like an orchestra producing a symphony,' he says. 'They cannot produce the full, beautiful effect on their own, so we need to consider the levels of every one.'

What is Conventional HRT?

HRT aims to alleviate the symptoms of menopause by replacing some of the hormones that women's bodies stop producing at menopause. Nearly all conventional

HRT formulas consist of either oestrogen alone, or oestrogen plus a synthetic type of progesterone called progestin. The oestrogen may be derived from plants or, if you are taking the continuous type of HRT, using conjugated equine oestrogens such as Premarin or prempro, from the urine of pregnant mares. These synthetic or horse hormones are supposed to be better absorbed than natural ones, but they do not act in exactly the same way as our own natural hormones, and many people believe they are not as beneficial. There are more than sixty different preparations of HRT made by different pharmaceutical companies and combined in varying proportions. Mostly they are delivered via a pill, patch or gel.

'Conventional HRT, although very successful by and large, is a mixed blessing, with side effects that tend to offset the benefits to some degree,' says Dr Sister. 'In part, this is because HRT entails the use of synthetic hormones, such as the progestins in Provera, or natural ones derived from horse urine. When I say natural, they are natural for horses, but not for humans.'

Cyclical HRT normally delivers oestrogen every day, plus a synthetic type of progestogen called progestin, to replace the natural hormone progesterone. This results in a bleed or 'period' after the progestogen phase. It is usually given to peri-menopausal women who are still having periods, even if they are naturally infrequent. Occasionally it is offered to women post-menopause who want to experience periods. (Why would you? Search us!)

Continuous HRT involves a daily dose of oestrogen and progestins. This prevents the womb lining building up so you don't have periods. Both can be given as a tablet, patch or implant.

Some women in peri-menopause opt instead for the Mirena intra-uterine device, which is a coil-like apparatus designed for use as a contraceptive. This releases tiny daily doses of levonorgestrel, a synthetic progestogen. It tends to stop periods, and some women love it as it boosts progesterone and acts as a birth control at the same time. Others experience quite severe side effects, including breakthrough bleeding, weight gain and acne. The Mirena can be combined with an oestrogen patch to better control menopausal symptoms.

Oestrogen alone can also be applied to the vagina as a cream, a pessary, a ring, or with an applicator for local symptoms such as dryness, especially during sex. Slow-release implants, which are inserted under the skin and replaced every six months, are also available.

As you can see, HRT has pros and cons that you will need to discuss with your doctor. But it's worth remembering that there is an alternative to conventional HRT, which offers all the benefits, but with a more individual approach. This is called bio-identical hormone therapy.

What Are Bio-Identical Hormones?

Dr Sister specializes in this alternative to conventional HRT, which he strongly believes is more effective, has fewer side effects and is even safer. So what are bio-identical hormones and why are they different from conventional HRT?

Bio-identical hormones are compounds that are usually derived from plants such as yams, which are created in the laboratory to be exact chemical copies of your own human hormones. The key thing that makes bio-identical hormones different from the oestrogens derived from horse urine or synthetic versions of progesterone is that they work in your body in exactly the same way as your own youthful hormones used to. It is vital to point out that this does not mean these are 'quack' medicines. They are not unregulated herbal concoctions, nor are they simple plant extracts or yam creams. They are an alternative to conventional HRT, but they are not 'alternative medicine' and they cannot be bought over the counter or on the internet, but must be prescribed by a doctor. In fact, many bio-identical hormones can be found in the doctor's bible, the *British National Formulary*, which is published under the authority of the Department of Health. Dr Sister prescribes hormones that have been medically approved, but he is very selective about which ones he uses.

He is also highly critical of the way that oestrogen alone is often given in conventional HRT to women who have had a hysterectomy. He says, 'If we need to balance oestrogen and progesterone before the menopause, there is absolutely no logic in not balancing them afterwards. Progesterone is essential to protect women's breasts, whether they have had a hysterectomy or not.'

The other difference with bio-identical hormone therapy is that doctors tend to supplement a much wider range of hormones, not just oestrogens and progesterone. This means it is far more bespoke, with each prescription designed for the individual's needs.

These are some of the key hormones that Dr Sister will consider supplementing using bio-identical hormones:

Progesterone

'An attractive alternative to conventional HRT is the use of natural progesterone,' says Dr Sister, 'particularly for women in peri-menopause.' Why? In the body, progesterone can be converted to all three types of oestrogen: oestrone, oestradiol and oestriol. It can also be converted to testosterone as needed.

Why take it? As we've already discussed, for women in their thirties and forties, a key cause of hormonal trouble is low progesterone, which is the first hormone to show a significant decline. While normal levels during your fertile years are something like 8–10 nanograms per millilitre, in menopause this drops to around 0.1–0.8 nanograms, which is pretty close to zero.

Progesterone deficiency can also be caused by chronic stress and polycystic ovary syndrome (PCOS), though conversely, a lack of progesterone can also trigger PCOS. It's a vicious circle.

Progesterone is a natural anti-depressant, promotes sleep and keeps you calm, so it can help with peri-menopausal irritation, anger jags and panic attacks, especially pre-menstrually. These symptoms are often caused by low progesterone.

Many peri-menopausal women also develop acne, especially on the neck, shoulders and back, and their hair can become thinner, too. Without enough progesterone, natural testosterone in the body converts to a potent form called DHT, which only adds to the acne and hair-loss misery.

Lack of progesterone and high levels of oestrogen together promote the growth of fibroids and may increase your risk of cancer.

Isn't it great to know there's a solution . . . ?

Oestrogen

When it comes to replacing oestrogen using bio-identical hormones, the key oestrogens are:

Oestriol

Because oestriol has been considered a by-product of another form of oestrogen and thus too weak to matter, it has been largely overlooked as a beneficial piece of the hormone pie. However, it appears oestriol can help reduce a variety of symptoms associated with peri-menopause and menopause, including:

- Hot flushes
- Vaginal dryness
- Decreasing bone density

Oestradiol

This is the primary sex hormone of childbearing women and it is responsible for female characteristics and sexual functioning. Also, oestradiol is important for women's bone health.

When levels fall at menopause, results can include thinning, dry, wrinkled skin; thinning bones; hot flushes; hair loss; urine infections; tiredness; memory loss; mood swings and exhaustion.

Testosterone

We all need testosterone for libido, energy, mental health and physical strength. If blood tests reveal low levels, supplementation may increase sexual frequency and pleasure. But it's not just about sex. Achy joints; thin, dry skin; brittle bones; fatigue and depression can also be signs of low testosterone levels. Testosterone helps rebuild muscle mass, reduce body fat, increase energy and improves the symptoms of rheumatoid arthritis. It can also increase the positive effects of oestrogen therapy and decrease depression, irritability, nervousness and insomnia. Like women, it's a multitasker.

Pregnenolone

This is a versatile little hormone! Pregnenolone can be turned into progesterone, or it can first be converted into DHEA or progesterone, then converted into either cortisol, testosterone or oestrogen. It tends to have a subtle effect on hormone balance, but may be particularly helpful for brain function and if you are under stress. Side effects, however, can include insomnia, anger and irritability, acne, hair loss and even heart palpitations. You can buy 50-mg capsules of pregnenolone over the counter, but it would be far safer to have it prescribed by a doctor.

Thyroid Hormones

If you feel fat, tired or weak, if you can't think straight, are depressed for no specific reason and feel cold when everyone else is warm and comfortable, you could well have a problem with your thyroid gland. Other symptoms that you aren't producing enough vital thyroid hormones include hair loss, dry or pale skin, brittle nails, muscle cramps, low blood pressure, high cholesterol and no libido.

The risk of developing diabetes is also increased, since thyroid hormones are needed to regulate blood sugar. Low thyroid hormones can also increase the risk of heart disease by raising levels of cholesterol and triglycerides and may cause high blood pressure.

The thyroid gland produces two main hormones: T4 (80 per cent) and T3 (20 per cent). When functioning properly, the body converts T4, which is mainly inactive, to T3 (triiodo thyroxin), which is the major active thyroid hormone. Think of T4 as crude oil – it needs to be converted to petrol before you can use it to fuel your car, or in this case, your body.

It's clear that some women with low thyroid levels are not being diagnosed fast enough, and they may not be getting the most effective treatments from their doctors either. For example, one study found that people with low thyroid levels felt best when taking T4 and T3, yet most doctors usually only prescribe T4. A GP can order a blood test for hypothyroidism, but if you want your level of T3 tested, it may be worth paying to see a private specialist for treatment. Dr Sister says, 'I always use a complete supplement with T4 and T3, and the dose is kept under constant review.'

DHEA

There is a single supplement that could help rebalance your hormones and make you feel much more youthful. Its name? DHEA. Actually, the full name is dehydroepiandrosterone, but you don't have to worry about that. You may not have heard of it, but it's actually your most abundant hormone when you are in your twenties. DHEA converts in the body into the sex hormones oestrogen, progesterone and testosterone as and when the body needs them. It seems to play an important role in creating and maintaining a lean body, too. The drop in levels of DHEA may even trigger the menopause itself, by causing levels of oestrogen to fall. While it's still not mainstream medicine, it seems that supplementing with a bio-identical form of DHEA derived from yams may have dramatic effects on some women in mid-life.

Dr Sister says, 'One interesting thing discovered recently by Italian researchers at the University of Modena and the University of Pisa is that DHEA can be helpful in enhancing the post-menopausal years in women. It appears to offer some of the same benefits as those of hormone replacement therapy.'

DHEA seems to boost libido, improve your immune system and could reduce your risk of diabetes and osteoporosis. It may also prevent bone loss, and even increase bone density. It seems to lower cholesterol levels, and stabilizes blood sugar and insulin. It can also reduce menopausal symptoms such as hot flushes. In the mid-nineties, researchers at the University of Southern California School of Medicine La Jolla did the first controlled human clinical trials of DHEA replacement therapy. The trial was small, but the results were startling: 85 per cent of women on DHEA said their wellbeing improved after taking DHEA, compared to only 5 per cent taking a placebo. Their immune systems improved, they were more relaxed and more resistant to stress.

Taking DHEA may even increase skin thickness and moisture, and decrease age spots. It almost sounds too good to be true! In general, DHEA is considered safe, but overdoses, or even smallish doses in women who are not deficient may have some reversible side effects, such as greasy hair and skin; acne on the face, scalp, chest and back, and unwanted facial hair. However, Susie has been taking DHEA for over ten years in 25-mg doses, and is terrified about stopping as she feels the results have been amazing!

DHEA is available on prescription only in the UK, but is available over the counter in many other countries.

Melatonin to Boost Natural Melatonin and Reduce Cortisol

Supplements of melatonin can be used as a natural way to help you get to sleep. Many of us swear by it to treat jet lag, and studies show that it helps you feel much more human! It is also a potent antioxidant. Many studies demonstrate that it shortens the time it takes to fall asleep, but this may be by minutes, not hours. It is particularly effective as we get older. It's been tested and found to help with cluster headaches, and one dose helps quell anxiety, irritability and cravings for up to ten hours if you are giving up smoking. It also naturally reduces cortisol.

How much should you take? For cluster headaches, you may need as much as 10 mg of melatonin at night. But for reducing anxiety when stopping smoking, and to help you sleep, 0.3 mg is an effective dose. You shouldn't take melatonin with alcohol, and too much can lead to extremely vivid nightmares and may also make you sleepy during the day.

Melatonin is freely available over the counter in the US, but is on prescription only in the UK.

More nutrients to help balance your hormones and make you feel fabulous:

5-Hydroxytryptophan (5-HTP) for Serotonin

5-HTP is a naturally occurring amino acid, which is necessary for the production of the 'happy hormone' serotonin and the sleep hormone melatonin. Several double-blind, placebo-controlled studies have shown that it may be effective as a treatment for depression. It may reduce appetite and help you feel fuller, so a supplement can even help you lose weight. 5-HTP also seems to have the potential to reduce anxiety, binge eating and insomnia.

A normal dose of 5-HTP ranges from around 50 to 400 mg. For depression, the normal dosage will involve taking a 50-mg capsule once to four times daily. You can buy 5-HTP over the counter. Side effects are rare and no risks have been identified, though some users complain of an upset stomach.

Amino Acids for Growth Hormone

As we sleep, the pituitary gland deep inside the brain is busy secreting growth hormone (GH). This is vital for tissue repair, muscle growth, healing, brain function, physical and mental health, bone strength, energy and metabolism. As with the other hormones, levels fall as we age. In fact, some specialists say the fall in GH is a primary factor in the ageing process. It causes reduced endurance, low sex drive, decreased bone density, decreased muscle mass and reduced cardiac function, blood sugar control, immunity and memory. But there's a problem. It's hard to measure how much GH we have in a blood test, as amounts fluctuate radically during the day. However, we can test levels of insulin-like growth factor-1 (IGF-1), which is a stable marker for GH.

Doctors must be cautious, though, as IGF-1 is made in the liver under the influence of GH, but if our liver is stressed by liver disease, insulin deficiency, low thyroid, or because we are ill or injured, levels of IGF-1 may fall, even though GH levels are normal.

If you have low IGF-1 without any obvious signs of liver stress, then you may have low GH. A supplement may seem to be the obvious answer, but there has been a move away from expensive, painful injections of GH, partly because these interfere with the body's own secretion of the hormone. Exercise, particularly weight training, boosts GH production by up to 20 per cent, but you can also take amino acids, which work to stimulate the pituitary to 'act younger' and make more natural GH. These include amino acids like L-arginine, ornithine, L-lysine, glutamine, methionine, cysteine, tyrosine and glycine. A simpler solution is the supplement YOUTH, which contains amino acids shown to raise levels of GH.

Magnesium

Do you know that around 70 per cent of women don't get enough magnesium in their diet? Yet this vital mineral is needed by every cell in the human body and is required for more than 300 biochemical reactions. It's vital for nerve and muscle function, regulates your heartbeat, keeps your bones strong and may prevent high blood pressure and heart disease. It controls glucose metabolism and deficiencies appear to make insulin resistance worse and could even increase the risk of Type 2 diabetes. It's also essential for the balance of a hormone called parathyroid hormone, which has the job of regulating the amount of calcium in the blood.

If you are chronically short of magnesium you will become, quite literally, sick and tired. Early symptoms of magnesium deficiency include loss of appetite, nausea and tiredness. If untreated you might develop muscle cramps and depression.

Magnesium can help you sleep, relax muscles and reduce corstisol levels. The EC RDA for adult women is 375 mg a day, and it's found in nuts, green vegetables, fortified grains, milk, beans and rice, but it's tricky to get enough in a modern diet with processed foods, hence the high deficiency levels.

Vitamins B12, Folic Acid and B6

These B vitamins play a vital part in producing several hormones and neurotransmitters that affect your mood, including dopamine, serotonin and melatonin. They also reduce levels of an amino acid called homocysteine, which circulates in the blood, though it's not known if this actually causes the problems or is just a signal for them – studies are ongoing. Homocysteine is linked with dementia, Alzheimer's, general loss of mental function and depression in older women.

The EC RDA of B6 is 1.4 mg, for folic acid 200 mcg and for B12, 2.5 mcg. However, evidence indicates that the latter is too low, and 6 mcg is a more effective yet safe dose of B12. In fact, in the US, older people are encouraged to take a B12 supplement and there's no evidence that higher levels are toxic. Though we don't recommend mega doses, B vitamins are usually very safe. To prevent macular degeneration of the eye, doses of 50 mg of B6 are prescribed, with 1,000 mcg of B12 and 2,500 mcg of folic acid. Delicious food sources of B vitamins include oily fish and seafood, beef, lamb, pork, green vegetables, peas, beans and yoghurt.

Vitamin C

Vitamin C is a bit of a wonder vitamin. It helps regulate thyroid hormone production and also reduces the amount of inflammatory histamine in the body. This may make vitamin C useful to treat allergies. It's also a powerful antioxidant and helps boost the immune system. Plus vitamin C is vital for the formation of collagen in the skin. A key feature of vitamin C is that it's a very powerful stress buster. Studies show that people under stress given a 1,000-mcg dose of vitamin C have far lower levels of cortisol, which we know is a hormone that is bad news for your weight, blood sugar, inflammation and immune system. The EU RDA recommended daily amount is 80 mg, but many experts feel this may be too low and that 100 mg is a more effective dose. You'll find it naturally in red peppers, broccoli, strawberries, oranges, melon, kiwi and cauliflower, so it's easy to get enough in food if you eat a healthy diet.

Selenium

Selenium controls thyroid functions. For a healthy metabolism, we need to make sure we give the thyroid everything it needs to operate well, and yet many women are deficient in selenium. Selenium is also a mood-booster. Studies indicate that low selenium causes depression, confusion, anger and anxiety. The EC RDA is 55 mcg and the highest food sources are shellfish, fish and, best of all, nuts. Just two brazil nuts will give you your daily selenium requirement. Make them dark chocolate brazils for a spot of extra magnesium.

Vitamin E

This vitamin boosts progesterone production, which can balance high oestrogen. Vitamin E is a great antioxidant for the skin, helps regulate vitamin A, reduces wrinkles and protects the skin from skin cancer and sunburn. Vitamin E may also help protect the brain from Alzheimer's and Parkinson's disease. Studies show that vitamin E may reduce PMS symptoms, including tender breasts, and during the menopause, a study showed daily supplements of vitamin E helped to slightly reduce both the frequency and severity of hot flushes. Vitamin E is measured in IUs and in mg. The EC RDA for vitamin E is 12 mg a day (around 22IU). High doses above 400 mg taken long-term should be avoided, as they may have side effects. To eat your vitamin E, choose almonds, sunflower seeds, olives, spinach and blueberries.

Vitamin D3

Vitamin D3 is different to other vitamins, because we don't have to eat it. Instead, we make nearly all our vitamin D in our bodies as a response to sunlight on our skin. When we get vitamin D, it is processed by the body into a hormone called calcitrol, which, among other things, regulates the amount of calcium in our blood, bones and gut and helps our cells communicate. Every cell in our body has a receptor for vitamin D. Low vitamin D is linked to eighteen auto-immune diseases, including asthma and multiple sclerosis, to cancers including breast cancer, and high blood pressure. Vitamin D switches on or off a staggering 900 genes, and affects over 2,000. It can also help maintain your strength and balance, and increasing evidence shows vitamin D deficiency causes pain and stiffness, especially in the joints. Supplements have been said to prevent pain. It's a fact that many people with unexplained back pain have a vitamin D deficiency – and fatigue. It has been known for women to think they have chronic fatigue syndrome when in fact they are just horribly low in vitamin D. It's impossible to state just how important this vitamin/hormone is, but it's estimated that up to half the women in the UK are vitamin D deficient, and this is despite the advice that we'll get enough just by exposing our SPF-free arms to the sun for ten to fifteen minutes a day during the summer. Given how much time we spend indoors and covered up, and how much, frankly, it rains, it's not surprising.

Medical advice now is that everyone needs some time in the sun – even if that's just a few minutes a day in the summer – without sunscreen. This doesn't mean you have to roast, and you should certainly never burn, but getting sunshine on your skin is very important – there's a reason it feels so good.

Food sources include oily fish, eggs, butter and milk,

but it's very difficult to get enough from food alone. It's estimated that even with a good diet, we could only get 10 per cent of our needs from the food we eat.

The alternative is a supplement. Strangely, there are two units of measurement for vitamin D. The recommended amount of vitamin D is just 400 IU, or 10 mcg, but our need for vitamin D increases with age – the Department of Health recommends people over 65 take a 10 mcg supplement every day – and many experts take much more than that. There are two forms of vitamin D as supplements: vitamin D2 and vitamin D3. Vitamin D3 is safer, more natural and more effective. Higher doses up to 2000 IU or 50 mcg a day have been found to be safe in studies. Indeed, it's roughly the amount generated when we expose our face and forearms to the sun at midday for half an hour in summer. In sunny countries, natural vitamin D levels are three times higher than in the UK, and many researchers in the field take 100 mg a day. It's very safe to take in higher doses, and as the sun doesn't come in a bottle, we'd recommend a supplement. Leah uses D3 in spray form, which is great for absent-minded or busy people as you carry it in your bag and use like a breath freshener (it's even minty!), but you can get a blood test to tell if you are deficient, which is the safest way to monitor your levels.

Vitamin K

Never heard of this one? That's fine, it doesn't get talked about much. But it's vital, especially as you get older. You know how important vitamin D3 is, especially for your bones? Well, vitamin K2 is a very clever nutrient that's vital for strong bones, protects against heart disease, stops you getting varicose veins, protects against broken and thread veins on the face and even makes you look younger and less wrinkly. How? Vitamin K2 controls calcium in the blood, directing it to your bones and teeth, while preventing it from ending up as calcium deposits in the arteries. After the menopause, low oestrogen levels mean the reverse starts to happen. And this may be made worse by a deficiency of K2. Studies at the University of York and the University of Copenhagen have shown that vitamin K2 deficiency is linked to decreased bone density and increased fracture risk, while supplementation with vitamin K2 reduces bone loss and fractures.

A supplement of vitamins D3 and K2 appears to be more effective at preventing bone loss than just one vitamin. In fact, it can actually increase your bone density. K2 may also prevent hardening of the arteries, keeping them as stretchy and elastic as a yoga devotee, and that's great for heart health.

It also seems to prevent insulin resistance by boosting levels of the hormone adiponectin, which makes cells sensitive to insulin. And because it prevents calcium stiffening up cells, it can even fight wrinkles. People with a genetic condition that causes low vitamin K are known to develop severe premature wrinkles, but K2 appears to keep our elastin fibres smooth and springy, which means fewer lines and less sagging.

So how do you get enough? There are two forms of vitamin K. K1, or phylloquinone, is found in leafy green vegetables such as lettuce, broccoli and spinach. This makes up around 90 per cent of the vitamin K in an average diet. Then there is K2, or menaquinone. This is synthesized from K1 by microflora in the gut, but is also found in meat, eggs, butter (especially butter from grass-fed cows) and fermented food products like cheese, yoghurt and pickles like sauerkraut.

Diet alone is often not enough to give us the optimum amount of K2. Unlike other fat-soluble vitamins, such as vitamins A, D and E, vitamin K can't be stored in the body, so we need a daily dose. It's vital to avoid evil trans fats, as they stop vitamin K from working, so ditch processed foods and cheap ready meals. It's also important to nurture the precious healthy flora of your gut, where most K2 is made. So follow the tips for healthy gut flora in the chapter on inflammation, and eat garlic, artichokes, leeks, bananas and onions, which are powerful prebiotics, containing a type of starch that feeds good bacteria. Also try probiotics, either in the form of special drinks or in natural live yoghurt, and don't take antibiotics unnecessarily – some conditions, such as colds and most ear infections, simply don't need them.

Case Study: Jessica Story

Jessica, fifty-four, arrived at Dr Sister's consulting rooms and slumped in a chair, exhausted. A chic, successful businesswoman in Jimmy Choo shoes, she explained she had been suffering from hot flushes and insomnia, but what really worried her was that four years ago a bone scan revealed she had osteopenia, an early form of the bone-thinning disease osteoporosis. She had been to see a hormone specialist and had been prescribed bio-identical hormones, but her symptoms had persisted and even got worse. Dr Sister was horrified that nobody had thought to re-test her bone density since the first scan, so he immediately sent her for a full blood test, plus a new bone scan. He soon discovered that her bones had deteriorated and that she needed a different balance of hormones. His prescription included a different form of oestrogen – oestriol – plus testosterone for her bones. One month later, a very different Jessica arrived for her follow-up appointment, with brighter skin and a twinkle in her eye. She told the doctor her hot flushes had disappeared and she didn't just feel renewed energy at work, but at home, too. More specifically, the testosterone had given her sex life a boost and her marriage was happier than ever. Jessica will continue to have her hormones and bone density monitored regularly.

Take Control!

- Hormone replacement therapy is shown to be safe for most women if taken at the right time, under the right supervision and at the right dosage. In fact, it dramatically cuts your risk of premature death and reduces your risk of dementia.
- The best time to replace hormones is when you notice changes associated with falling hormones

and for the ten years after the menopause, but longer if you need it and are under medical supervision.

- Progesterone is the first hormone to show a steep decline, even before the menopause.
- After the menopause, oestrogen therapy with other hormones can dramatically reduce menopausal symptoms.
- Bio-identical hormones are closer to your body's natural hormones.
- Hormone therapy is not for everyone and should be tailored to you as an individual.
- If you can't take hormones, other supplements used together can help adjust hormone imbalances.
- Supercharging your diet can be more effective than taking supplements for most nutrients and is always safe.
- It's impossible to get enough vitamin D from your diet alone. You need sunshine or a supplement, ideally both.
- If you have symptoms of tiredness, depression, aches and pains, then testing for deficiencies of certain nutrients such as iron and vitamin D should be offered.
- Get your thyroid tested if you notice any of the symptoms of hypo- or hyper-thyroidism.

'And the beauty of a woman, with passing years only grows!'
Audrey Hepburn

12. Take Control: Getting the Medical Care You Deserve

What should you do if you want to try hormone therapy? Here is some general advice on getting the best from your medical care.

Pick the Right Doctor

If you now feel hormone replacement is right for you, then your first step is to make an appointment, either with your GP or with a specialist hormone medical doctor. Beware of practitioners who use titles like 'naturopathic doctor' or 'homeopathic doctor'. These aren't real doctors at all, so cannot legally prescribe hormones. It's likely they will just give you overpriced vitamins and other over-the-counter supplements.

Be Assertive

We know from our friends and our experiences that it's not always easy to get the best treatment for hormone issues, and you may need to change GPs to get appropriate treatment. Red flags that you won't be treated well include being told, 'It's normal at your age to feel X or Y.' Remember, age is not a disease, and age alone cannot account for any symptoms. There is always a reason for any symptoms you suffer at any age, and a good doctor will help you find that reason. We believe that if your doctor ever says, 'It's your age,' then you should change doctor! We've also seen shocking signs in doctors' waiting rooms saying, 'One Symptom Per Appointment'. This is a sign that your doctor is simply not interested in treating you as a whole person, and it's also potentially dangerous, as very few conditions have only one symptom! We'd advise steering clear of surgeries where you see this sign. (See Hannah's story at the end of this chapter for an example of someone who was nearly killed by a doctor who thought this way.)

Keep a Hormone Diary

Whichever path you chose, before you see a doctor, keep a hormone diary for a few weeks or months. Note when your last period was, and any physical or mental symptoms you have noticed. If you are having hot flushes, try to keep a note of how often you get them, when you get them and how severe they are. This will give your doctor an idea of what your key concerns are.

Dr Sister will always perform a blood test before offering treatment. If you see a private hormone doctor, they will normally ask you to have tests to check your levels of the following hormones and health markers:

- Triglycerides
- Cholesterol: total, HDL, LDL
- DHEA sulphate
- Vitamin D
- The thyroid hormones TSH, T4 and T3

- FSH
- Oestradiol
- Progesterone
- Testosterone
- Luteinizing hormone

These tests, if done at a private lab, will cost around £400.

- Talk through the pros and cons with your doctor. There are few cases where you absolutely cannot take hormones of any kind.
- HRT dosage should be individualized. Ask your doctor why that particular dosage or combination of hormones is perfect for you.
- Expect regular reviews of your treatment to ensure it meets your changing needs. This should happen every few months as you settle into treatment, and then at least annually afterwards.
- Go back to your doctor if your symptoms aren't resolved or get worse. It can take a long time to get your hormones balanced.

Hormone Therapy Q&A

Q: Can I get pregnant on HRT?
A: Yes. The type of oestrogen used in HRT is not as strong or powerful as that used in the Pill. If you don't want to get pregnant, and are using HRT, you should use non-hormonal contraception for two years after

your last period if you started the menopause before fifty, and one year if you are over fifty. Some hormonal treatments for peri-menopause are also types of contraception. If you would still like a baby, but have menopausal symptoms, you should visit your doctor or a fertility specialist before taking any hormones.

Q: I've had breast cancer but sex is painful. Can I take hormones?

A: This is a difficult one and you will need to talk to your doctor. Normally you wouldn't be offered HRT, but vaginal oestrogen therapy in the form of a ring or gel is a possible option for you.

Q: I've had cervical cancer. Can I take HRT?

A: It's not contra-indicated and there is no evidence that HRT will harm you but, as always, you need to talk about your individual risks with your doctor.

Q: I'm a year into menopause. I'd like to stop my hot flushes but I like not having a monthly bleed. Will HRT mean my periods start up again?

A: No. Continuous HRT, which is offered on the NHS after you have gone a year without periods, will not give you periods.

Q: I'm sixty. Replacing my hormones has changed my life, but my GP wants me to stop taking HRT. Are there limits on how long I'm allowed to take it?

A: No. If you still have symptoms, the benefits of hormone therapy usually outweigh the risks. You are entitled to see another GP if you aren't happy with your treatment.

Q: When is the best time to take HRT?

A: Usually it's best to start it before you are sixty. If you want to take it after this to control symptoms, then talk to your doctor. It's reasonable to start on a low dose to see how you feel. A patch is the safest way to take HRT at this age.

Q: I had an early menopause at thirty-five and have been on HRT for ten years. Is this safe?

A: For the sake of your health, it is extremely important that you replace your hormones if you have an early natural menopause or have had your ovaries removed. It is best to take hormones at least until the average age of menopause, which is fifty-two, and ideally beyond.

Q: Why does my doctor want me to use a patch for HRT? It's such a faff and I'd prefer a pill.

A: We know how you feel, but any method of delivering hormones that puts them directly into the blood-stream, where hormones belong, instead of being 'digested' via the liver, is more natural, safer and less likely to cause side effects. So creams, gels and patches are usually preferred to pills.

Q: How soon can I expect my symptoms to go away?

A: Hot flushes and sweats usually improve two to three weeks after starting treatment; other symptoms may take a little longer. Maximum benefits are usually felt after three to four months.

Q: I'm on HRT but still have symptoms, such as tired-ness and brain fog. Why aren't they getting better?

A: Possibly you need a different type of hormone therapy, perhaps with some testosterone. However, you may also need to think about lifestyle changes. Less stress, more sleep, more exercise and a healthy diet can work wonders. But you know that by now, right?

Q: What are the side effects of HRT?

A: You could get breast tenderness, nausea, leg cramps and some spotting. If they don't wear off within a couple of weeks, your doctor should adjust your dose or give you a different sort of HRT. Often side effects are due to an intolerance of non bio-identical progestogens. Bio-identical progesterone is better tolerated and often has fewer unwanted side effects.

Q: Will I put on weight?

A: HRT rarely causes weight gain. It is more likely to help you lose weight, especially belly fat. Some women do gain weight, but this may be due to bloating as your body adjusts to the hormones.

Q: When should I bleed and how long should it be for?w

A: Most women on a cyclical HRT have a four- to seven-day bleed, although it may be shorter. Women using continuous HRT may have irregular bleeding in the early months.

Q: If I couldn't take the contraceptive pill, can I take HRT?

A: Yes, unfortunately there is a misunderstanding about how HRT differs from the contraceptive pill.

Q: What about HRT and osteoporosis?

A: If you start HRT at around the time your periods finish you will help to prevent the onset of osteoporosis, a condition in which bones become very fragile and often fracture when older. Studies have shown that five years' use of HRT is associated with halving the risk of a hip fracture.

Q: What happens when HRT is stopped?

A: When HRT is stopped bone density declines. This is normally at the same rate as immediately after the menopause. However, the rapid loss experienced at this time is delayed by the length of time a woman takes HRT.

Q: I'm fifty-two and feel fine, but my mother and grand-mother both had severe osteoporosis. Should I take HRT?

A: You should ask your doctor for a bone-density test or you could take one privately so you know how healthy your bones are, but generally, hormone therapy is recommended for preserving your bones and preventing osteoporosis, and it's best to start when you are under sixty.

Q: I've had a blood clot in my leg before. Is HRT safe for me?

A: Oral HRT does increase the risk of clots. However, the risk is highest with oral HRT and synthetic progestogens. Testing to discover the reason for the dot, such as genetic reasons, can help establish your risk levels. It may be possible to take HRT via a patch and using bio-identical progesterone. Again, you must discuss the risks with your doctor.

Q: I'm interested in trying testosterone as part of my HRT. Can I get this on the NHS?

A: We're sorry to say this may be difficult. Specific testosterone patches for women are no longer available in the UK. They were withdrawn for commercial reasons, not health ones, which indicates that few doctors were prescribing them even when they were licensed. If you are a year into the menopause, you may consider asking for Livial tablets. These contain itibolone, which is a synthetic steroid that breaks down to compounds that act in a similar way to oestrogen, progesterone and testosterone. It helps prevent bone loss. If you are peri-menopausal or would prefer a bio-medical option, some GPs will prescribe Testogel, a bio-identical testosterone gel that is usually only available for men, but can be given to women in smaller doses. If your GP refuses, there are a number of private clinics offering bio-identical testosterone replacement.

Case Study: Hannah's Story

At the age of fifty-three, out of the blue, Hannah, a fitness teacher and personal trainer, started to suffer terrible aches and pains and found herself taking paracetamol almost every day. Concerned, she visited her GP only to be told, 'It's your age. You're doing too much.' But for Hannah, fitness was her job and paid her mortgage. Also, she didn't want to do less. Movement was her life. So she simply took more painkillers, though never more than the daily dose recommended on the packet.

Then something frightening started to happen. She found herself collapsing in the street as her muscles inexplicably gave way. She went to her GP. The sign on the wall said, 'One Symptom Per Appointment', so this time she raised the issue of the falls. The doctor barely looked at her. 'It's your age. It's normal for older women to have falls.' Soon Hannah started suffering symptoms that weren't just physical. She became muddled in her thinking. She found it hard to make decisions. And what she didn't realize for a long time was that she was becoming horribly, terrifyingly depressed.

Slowing down, said her doctor, was 'just normal' for her age. 'People get depressed as they get older.' Then a crisis happened. All those painkillers practically burned a hole in her stomach and she collapsed with internal bleeding. Even more scarily, when she got to hospital, they found her kidneys were failing from taking too many painkillers.

She was in a terrible state, but ironically, this was her lucky break, because then and only then did the doctors do a very simple, inexpensive blood test that discovered the reason for all her symptoms. Her thyroid had pretty much stopped producing any hormones whatsoever. No wonder her body was in meltdown. Now, five years later, Hannah has fortunately recovered. She takes one tiny tablet of the synthetic thryroid hormone thyroxine a day and is still teaching classes, and loves travelling.

It took her a while to get the right dose, and it still needs adjusting from time to time, but she has got her life back. She says, 'How many other women are seeing their GPs complaining of suffering from fatigue, aches and depression, and being fobbed off or, perhaps even worse, put on lifelong anti-depressants, without a single blood test? Who gave up exercising, gave up on life and died early? I've discovered that deficiencies in thyroid hormones are very common in older women. I think every women in mid-life who presents with symptoms like mine should automatically have their thyroid tested. And don't hesitate to change a doctor who blames your age or isn't interested in hearing about *all* your symptoms. I could have died. I feel so lucky to be here.'

Take Control!

- Symptoms you think may be purely hormonal may instead be connected to stress or lifestyle issues, such as diet or lack of exercise. If your blood tests come back normal, your symptoms may be best treated by paying attention to your general health.
- Blood tests are vital, but they are the start of the process, not the end of it.
- As hormones are very powerful, they can have side effects if the dosage is wrong.
- Insist on a thyroid function test and vitamin D tests before you take anti-depressants.
- If your doctor won't give you tests, or insists your symptoms are 'just your age', find another doctor. We really mean this.
- Hormone supplementation should always be carefully monitored by a doctor who is trained and experienced. This isn't something you can take on as a DIY project.

'I married an archaeologist, because the older I grow, the more he appreciates me.'
Agatha Christie

13. Take Control: Looks

Future Perfect: How the Latest Beauty Technology Can Reverse the Visible Effects of Ageing

We all want to look our best at any age. While we don't want, or expect, to look nineteen again, we know that looking prettier, healthier and younger, or simply 'good for our age', has a powerful effect on our self-esteem and confidence. Research shows that if you look more youthful, people will react towards you as if you are younger, which can affect your physical health. As we explained in Chapter 2, simply seeing a younger reflection in the mirror can have a dramatic effect on your hormones and your health.

And it's not just about looking younger. Some of us feel that as we age our faces change in ways that are normally associated with emotions such as anger (the frown line between our brows that won't go away) or sadness (the droop to our lips), which we simply don't feel. So the face we present to the world – and that other people react to – doesn't reflect our true personalities. This is why Leah has Botox® between her brows to nix her frown line.

She has pictures of herself as a toddler, frowning furiously, so she got a line in her late twenties. Now she doesn't. She's had laser treatment and IPL (Intense Pulsed Light) to reduce tiny red veins and brighten her skin. Susie swears by regular sessions of PRP (Platelet-Rich Plasma therapy), aka Dracula therapy, to plump up her face and make her skin radiant. She also embraces IPL plus twice yearly microdermabrasion. They aren't embarrassed by these interventions any more than they are embarrassed about the fact that they both colour their hair.

In fact, more and more of us are seeking out ways to look better, and increasingly calling on doctors to help us. The traditional facelift is no longer the first option. In fact, it is often the very last resort for women with a lot of loose skin. Instead, there are a host of new non-invasive, non-surgical, high-tech procedures that can delay and even reverse the signs of ageing, tightening skin, restoring fullness, relaxing wrinkles and improving the texture of your skin. This leaves you looking fresh and vital, with a face that reflects the way you really feel inside.

So What's Really Making You Look Older?

Hormonal changes in mid-life and beyond definitely affect your looks. The first sign? Not wrinkles, but loss of volume. In the first five years after the menopause you lose 30 per cent of your collagen (the fibres that give substance to skin). Production of elastin, which keeps skin stretchy and bouncy, also starts to decline. This means skin starts to lose its moisture, structure, thickness and firmness.

But skin isn't the only thing that thins. Hormone-induced bone loss makes your skull literally shrink, and your facial fat starts to shift, too, so that you become hollow around the eyes and cheeks, creating jowls and a gaunt appearance. This is why, though a lithe body is youthful, after the age of forty, weight loss of more than 10 lbs can make you look older, while a few extra pounds makes you look younger. Fat is a natural filler!

Hormone replacement can help reverse skin ageing. A study in the *British Medical Journal* showed that post-menopausal women who had oestrogen and testosterone therapy had 48 per cent more collagen than women who hadn't had hormone therapy. A University of Vienna study in post-menopausal women found that oestrogen improved skin elasticity and firmness after just six months of treatment, and both wrinkle depth and pore size decreased by more than 60 per cent. This can make women look around four years younger than they otherwise would.

Of course, external factors also contribute to ageing. A poor diet, lack of skin-friendly vitamins, bad fats and sugary carbs will leave skin looking grey and old. Smoking, too, is a disaster for skin, activating genes responsible for a skin enzyme called collagenase, which breaks down collagen in the skin. It also reduces blood flow to the skin, which is why smokers have more wrinkles and tend to have a greyish pallor, rather than the kind of rosy glow we all want. In fact, it's been found that every ten years of smoking adds two and a half years to your appearance.

Stress and unhappiness can also add years to your appearance. A plastic surgeon tracked the faces of his patients over many years and found that a stressful event could accelerate ageing by up to five years in just one.

Divorce or illness in particular made women look visibly older by around eighteen months, partly due to the effects of cortisol.

The final major factor is sun damage. UVA rays cause elastin, another fibrous skin component, to reorient itself from its normal position to one that's parallel to the surface of your skin, where it begins to reproduce in unusually high amounts. The presence of this abnormal elastin causes a secretion of enzymes called metalloproteinases. These enzymes destroy collagen and elastin by, in effect, chopping them into small pieces, making skin saggy and baggy, so that it falls into folds and wrinkles.

UVA rays also trigger abnormal melanin production, which causes brown spots. The best prevention? Keep your skin out of the sun, don't burn and wear a broad-spectrum SPF of at least 30 in strong sunshine, and SPF15 the rest of the time.

Broad spectrum means it protects against UVB, which burns, and UVA, which ages you. Look for the letters UVA in a circle, which indicates good UVA protection, or the PA+++ symbol, which was developed in Asia to rate UVA protection. PA+++ is more protective than P+.

New formulations also protect against infrared, which heats the skin and dilates tiny blood vessels, making redness and rosacea skin conditions worse.

Micronized powder formulations can be a great way to layer on sunscreen during the day, especially if you wear make-up that would be ruined by a cream. An antioxidant serum containing vitamin C, or a mix of vitamins A, E and C, worn underneath, will boost the effectiveness of your sunscreen. Both Susie and Leah have a confession here: 'We both love the sun. We enjoy the feeling of warmth on our skin' – warmth is a proven anti-depressant – 'and enjoy the hormone and serotonin boost that warmth and light give us, and we need that vitamin D boost. We love the lift that bright light gives to our mood' – so important for melatonin production, too – 'but even if we sneak in a bit of sunbathing, we take great care never to burn, and always to keep our faces out of the way of those damaging rays.'

This advice ties in with that of the major health organizations. The British Association of Dermatologists, Cancer Research UK, Diabetes UK, the Multiple Sclerosis Society, the National Heart Forum, the National Osteoporosis Society and the Primary Care Dermatology Society all suggest going out in the middle of the day for a few minutes without sunscreen while exposing as much of your body as possible. You should not redden your skin or burn. Bikinis optional.

Treatments to Roll Back the Years

Once you've got your lifestyle, your hormones and your nutrition right, you will find you naturally age much more slowly and you should start to look healthier and glowing. A good antioxidant serum and a hydrating moisturizer will help slow the development of wrinkles and keep skin protected. Prescription retinol-based creams from a doctor or dermatologist have been proven to thicken, refine and smooth skin, thereby reversing ageing to some degree, though they can also be irritating. Treatments with a cosmetic doctor can also work wonders to create a more youthful look. The future of anti-ageing is bright. Only five years ago, even ultrasound and radio frequency weren't used for skin tightening, but now there are a host of new treatments available.

Our view? Less is definitely more, and remember, no procedure is entirely risk or side-effect free. Ensure you only ever get injected, needled or lasered by a trained expert, ideally a doctor. Never, ever allow a non-medic to inject Botox or fillers. The best way to find someone is by recommendation. Do you like the way your friend looks? Does she look fresh, rather than waxy or frozen? Does she say her doctor will listen to her concerns and fix anything that she doesn't like? Then you might have found the right man – or woman – for you. As for finding the right procedure for your problems, your doctor can suggest an anti-ageing plan for your concerns, but here's our guide to what's out there:

Chemical Peels

For superficial wrinkles, age spots, dull skin, large pores and mild acne scarring, a chemical peel can break up the 'glue' that holds the upper layers of skin cells together, so they painlessly slough off, causing new, fresh skin to be generated. The degree of peeling depends on the peeling agent. New types of peel penetrate the skin, so new skin is created in the deeper layers, emerging naturally with no actual peeling on the surface. Most peels are not painful, though acid peels may sting as they are applied. Do discuss thoroughly with your doctor.

Fillers

You know how ageing makes you lose volume in your mid face? The best way to replace it is with fillers. Yes, it can look overdone – the infamous pillow effect – but cleverly used fillers can give a fresh, youthful, happy appearance. Adding a little volume to gaunt faces also makes skin more taut – like blowing up a deflated balloon – so wrinkles and folds, such as those between the nose and mouth, disappear.

The safest fillers are made with hyaluronic acid, and these last from four months to a year, depending on their density, so if you hate the effect, you know it will wear off and you can even have hyaluronic acid dissolved, using a special antidote. Other fillers contain microspheres of calcium hydroxylapatite (Radiesse®), or polycapronolactone (Ellansé™), and these tend to last longer. They also dissolve naturally after around twelve to twenty-four months, but can't be reversed any earlier. Fat transfer is growing in popularity as new techniques and the use of stem-cell-enriched fat transfers mean that transplanted fat is more stable and lasts longer, but it can't ever be reversed. Fat injected around the eyes and upper face can be risky. And if you gain weight, the fat in your face will balloon.

You really should avoid permanent artificial fillers, as these have much higher risks of complications, and if you don't like the effect, you're stuck with it, like, um, for ever. Fillers can also be used very effectively on hands, making veiny old claws look like plump young paws. Fillers are medical treatments, not beauty treatments. Complications from wrong fillers or the wrong hands can include necrosis, which is when the skin literally dies and rots on your face, or even permanent blindness. A good knowledge of anatomy is essential. Always pick a trained doctor, dentist or nurse with plenty of experience.

Botulinum Toxin

It gets a bad press, but Botox® definitely works. Injections of this highly purified protein work to stop nerve impulses passing between muscles so they 'relax'. It's incredibly well tested, has been around for over twenty years in cosmetic medicine and even longer in conventional medicine, so it's extremely safe.

What's the difference between Botox® and hair dye? As we often say, they both make you look younger, but one is made with dangerous chemicals that can kill you and the other is Botox®! Our wrinkles are the result of repeated expressions, so Botox® can prevent as well as treat lines. Used between the brows it works wonders on frown lines, can reduce forehead tramlines and lift eyebrows.

Many doctors now use it on the lower face to reduce jowls, lift the corners of the mouth and soften neck bands. Injections into the jaw can even be used to stop tooth-grinding – Leah swears by this after years of being a tooth-grinder – and a happy side effect is a narrower, less square jawline.

Not everyone loves the look and feel of Botox®, though, so ask for a low dose to start with (a good doctor will always offer a follow-up appointment) and remember Botox® wears off in about three to six months. A bad effect, such as eyebrow droop – unfortunately this can happen – usually wears off sooner. Plenty of women are addicted to how it makes them look and feel, and in tests, a new zinc-based supplement called Zytaze® makes Botox® last around 30 per cent longer, making it a better bargain.

Botox is a prescription drug, which must be prescribed and overseen by a doctor, dentist or a nurse who is qualified to prescribe. Ensure the person wielding the syringe is one of these.

Laser Resurfacing

Lasers can be used to vaporize skin, and this is an effective treatment for badly wrinkled, sun-damaged skin. The depth of the laser resurfacing depends on the doctor and the treatment he recommends. Some can leave you looking like a burns victim, and it can hurt, despite local anaesthetic, while others are less invasive.

Fractional Resurfacing

Fractional treatments with lasers create tiny, microscopic holes in the skin, so only about 30 per cent of the surface skin is actually damaged for speedy healing and minimum downtime, while a healing response under the surface means your body creates new collagen and elastin. It's proven to be effective for skin tightening, reducing wrinkles and scars as well as pore size and making skin more even, smooth and radiant. The holes can be made by lasers or, more recently, by tiny needles that pass a radio-frequency energy current into the skin.

IPL or Photofacial

Intense Pulsed Light treatments can stimulate new collagen, and are particularly effective at removing brown and red pigments and treating tiny red veins in the face. These treatments feel like the face is being spattered by hot fat, but they're usually over very quickly. In the right hands, there is no actual injury to the skin, so there is no downtime. As with laser treatments, these must be performed by an experienced, trained specialist to avoid possible side effects, such as burning and pigment loss.

Photo-rejuvenation with LED Lights

Finally, a painless treatment! LED facials use light to improve the skin. Blue light can help kill acne bacteria, while red light reduces inflammation and gently boosts collagen. You are likely to need several treatments. LED facials are often used as part of other treatments as they can calm inflamed skin.

PRP Platelet-Rich Plasma Therapy

This treatment uses the clear part of your own blood, called plasma, which contains natural growth factors, to heal and regenerate. The plasma is then enriched with vitamins and amino acids, photoactivated and re-injected into the skin to stimulate repair. It leaves skin plump and subtly rejuvenated, and there is no risk of rejection or side effects as it is your own blood. This is Susie's favourite treatment.

Facial Needling

This treatment uses a spiked roller, or device that creates tiny wounds all over the skin, which stimulate a healing response and the formation of new collagen, elastin and blood vessels, so that skin looks plumper and more radiant. You'll usually be given a local anaesthetic cream to numb the skin, but it can still be quite painful.

Microdermabrasion

This treatment uses tiny particles that pass through a vacuum tube to gently scrape away the ageing skin and stimulate new cell growth. More of a facial than other non-surgical treatments, a course of treatments can still help decongest blocked pores, brighten skin and reverse skin damage, mild acne scarring and fine lines. Not suitable for some sensitive skin types. Hydrafacials, which infuse the skin with serums at the same time as exfoliating, are a gentler version of microdermabrasion. In Susie's spa the therapists recommend no more than three microdermabrasion treatments a year, as it can thin the skin and too much can create inflammation, which is ageing. And this is the reverse of what we want to do.

Carboxytherapy

Injections of carbon dioxide gas (CO_2) are a surprisingly effective way of tackling stretch marks, cellulite and dark eye bags. The needle stings a bit, and the bubbly sensation of the gas passing through the skin is odd, but not painful.

Leah says it reduced her post-pregnancy stretch marks quite dramatically. 'They pretty much disappeared, and I was very sceptical.' You can bruise, though not everyone does, so please be aware of this and allow for some downtime.

Non-Surgical Fat Loss

From cold lasers to freezing fat, there are a huge number of treatments out there to reduce fat without scalpels. Increasingly, even surgeons are turning to these non-invasive, scar-free methods.

Popular treatments include cryolipolysis, which literally freeze fat cells to death; and other treatments which claim to destroys fat cells with ultrasonic waves, as well as a cold laser treatment that claims to open up fat cells and empty them. Yet another is a combination of radio-frequency magnetic waves, ultrasound and light therapy and laser diodes to destroy fat cells and tighten skin. Some technologies, such as ultrasound and cryolipolysis, destroy fat cells permanently. Others empty fat cells. They work, but not if you indulge in too much chocolate cake with cream immediately afterwards!

All the various technologies have good science behind them, but none will make a fat person thin, so they're really for people at a healthy weight and size, but with lumps and bumps that bother them.

Future Technologies to Watch

Stem-cell technology is very exciting. Since fat cells contain adult stem cells – 10,000 more than in bone marrow – their use for facial rejuvenation is being explored and tested. For example, if stem cells from fat can turn into skin structure, they could be used to make a person look younger by adding volume to depressed facial areas. It may also be possible to use stem cells to reduce scarring, for sports injuries, arthritis, arthrosis and thyroid conditions.

Though these treatments are new and still being researched, some claim to trigger stem-cell renewal of bone, fat and skin, but so far the results have been unreliable, though the technology is progressing fast.

The very newest fat-fighting treatment uses injections of a naturally derived chemical called deoxycholate to destroy fat. It is tipped to be most useful for double chins but can also used for the body.

Supplements to Make You Look Younger

There is growing evidence that nutritional supplements can actually reverse skin ageing, boosting collagen, reducing wrinkles and patchy pigment as well as making skin thicker, smoother and more radiant. But don't expect miracles. A 30 per cent reduction in wrinkle depth is definitely worth having, but it will still leave you with 70 per cent of your wrinkles!

Some ingredients to look out for in effective skin supplements are marine plant extracts, isoflavones from soya, powerful antioxidants derived from plant extracts such as lycopene, carotenoids, white-tea and grape-seed extracts, superoxide dismutase, vitamin E, vitamin C – which your body needs to make collagen – and omega-3 fatty acids.

Can Skincare Help?

When it comes to preventing wrinkles, it seems a good moisturizer and sunscreen really can help. In research published in the *British Journal of Dermatology*, women were studied over eight years. If a woman had dry skin at twenty-eight, her wrinkles would have increased by 52 per cent by the time she reached thirty-six. But if the skin was kept hydrated and protected from the sun, wrinkles only increased by 22 per cent.

For wrinkles that have already formed, the most proven treatment is a prescription retinoic acid, such as tretinoin, which can reduce wrinkles, pigmentation and skin roughness. Creams containing up to 10 per cent vitamin C have also been proven to improve skin texture, wrinkles, pigment and hydration.

Vitamin C becomes ineffective when exposed to light, so when choosing a vitamin C product it's important to pick one in opaque packaging. It must have a pH of 3.0 or lower to be effective.

Niacinamide, a derivative of vitamin B3, has also been proven to reduce wrinkles, blotchiness, skin redness and yellowing. There is also evidence to suggest peptides and glucosamines can be effective at rejuvenating skin and, in the case of glucosamines, in evening out pigment for a brighter tomorrow.

And the most painless ways to drop a few years? Longer eyelashes can take an average of six years off your looks. Try a peptide serum to grow them, and a great mascara to highlight them. Lash extensions can be an instant eye-opener, but make sure you get good-quality ones, using glue that isn't too harsh.

Finally, did you know that your smell changes as you age? Don't worry, the body scent of older women was actually judged as more pleasant and subtle than that of younger women, but most people could correctly say if a woman was older than forty just by her smell! Turn back the clock by wearing citrus fragrances. In one study, men thought women who smelled of grapefruit were six years younger than they really were. That's almost as much as a full facelift, so spritz away the years.

Take Control!

- Get a great skin regime. Cleanse effectively, moisturize regularly, use an antioxidant serum and be careful to avoid ingredients that irritate or inflame your skin. For serious problems, see a dermatologist or cosmetic doctor.
- Botox® is safe, but as with all injectables, seek out a qualified medical practitioner.
- New technologies can rejuvenate skin, help with pigmentation and help reduce fat.
- Skincare supplements can help, as well as a good diet.
- Remember, less is more.

'Nature gives you the face you have at twenty; it is up to you to merit the face you have at fifty.'
Coco Chanel (1883–1971)

14. Take Control: Drop a Dress Size

Dr Sister's No-Deprivation, No-Hunger, Fast Fat-Loss Plan for a Healthier, More Youthful Body

As we've already said, you don't have to be skinny to be healthy, but as women of a certain age, we know that keeping our weight under control makes us feel good. A few extra pounds here and there can add up to stones as the years go by, and that really changes the way you look and feel. Suddenly your clothes don't fit, and you feel heavy and less inclined to go to that yoga class or head out for a run. You don't like what you see in the mirror, so you stop looking. If you aren't eating well and keeping active, you might even start to worry about your health. You might actively want to lose weight, and that's where this medically approved, hormone-balancing plan comes in.

Dr Sister has been helping women of all ages successfully lose weight for many years. As a hormone and anti-ageing specialist, he has devised this plan particularly for women in mid-life. It's designed to be simple and filling, so you don't get hungry and stressed. It's not calorie controlled, so it keeps your hormones in balance and your mood elevated, and it's designed to reduce insulin surges and help you lose fat, while protecting your lean muscle.

Typically, you can lose around 4–5 lbs in the first week

on this diet, and 1–2 lbs every week after that. But there's no point obsessing about the scales, because you can weigh more and look leaner if you lose fat but gain muscle. So remember, exercise is key, as it will help ensure the weight you lose is fat, not muscle.

Dr Daniel Sister has studied the science of food and hormones for decades and he says, 'The key to taking charge of our weight again is not by reducing the amount we eat, but changing what we eat, the time we eat and how we combine foods.' Here's how to eat as much as you want in terms of quantity, but still melt away fat.

This is not a calorie-controlled diet. Spending your life counting calories is like spending it in prison, and it's point-less. When we start cutting calories and getting hungry, our metabolisms, which remember are already on a go-slow, shift into an even lower gear. And to make things worse, our levels of brain dopamine fall, so we seek out fatty, sugary food to get a pleasure hit. We sleep badly so our hunger hormones soar and our body makes a hormone called reverse transcriptase. This slows the metabolism, making you sleepy, tired and keeping you fat. All in all, if you cut calories, getting hungry and regaining weight is pretty much guaranteed. So how can you lose weight with-out slashing your calorie intake? Easy. First, forget anything you have read about excess calories making us fat – the human body is a lot more complicated than that. Not all calories are created equal. Consuming 100 calories of pro-tein will not have the same effect on your body as 100 calories of carbs or fat. This means that with this plan you can eat well, even glamorously. A glass of wine and nibbles can be part of your life again. So say goodbye to starvation, and say hello to pleasure.

Why Fat is a Hormone Issue

A baby is born with around 5–6 billion fat cells. During childhood and in our teens we can gain extra fat cells if we are overweight, but in adulthood, our number of fat cells stays very stable, even if we put on weight. Surprised? But fat cells aren't always the same. They can literally be blown up like balloons, which is what makes us look bigger, and this process is driven by hormones, in particular, insulin.

When we eat sugar or carbs, these both convert to glucose in the body. High levels of glucose in our blood are dangerous, so insulin takes away all the glucose we don't burn off immediately as energy, and turns it into a substance called glycogen. Insulin then tucks this away in the liver and muscles to use as energy. However, if the glycogen storage systems are overwhelmed by the amount of glucose in the blood, insulin can turn all the glucose into fat, and store it in the fat cells. The more sugar and insulin we have in our bodies, the more fat is stored in the adipocytes – fat cells – and the fatter we look.

As long as our fat stays safely tucked away in our fat cells below the skin, we tend to stay healthy – even if we can't get our skinny jeans on – but if we gain more weight than our fat cells can cope with, we start to lay down fat in our abdomen and organs, such as the liver. And this is really bad news for our health.

Taking control of our insulin levels is therefore

absolutely vital if we want to lose fat. And the best way to tame our insulin levels is not to change the amount we eat, or the number of calories we eat; instead it's all about changing the type of food we eat. To see why, let's look at the four major food elements, and what they do to our hormones and our bodies.

Carbs: The Key to Hormonally Healthy Weight Loss

Carbohydrates come in two forms: sugars, which are found in sweet foods, including fruit, and starchy carbs, such as wheat, rice, beans, potatoes and even some green vegetables. In the body, both turn to glucose.

We like carbs because they taste good and fill us up, but this fullness is an illusion. When we eat carb-containing food – more specifically processed white carbs and sugar – they set up a massive hormone surge. Carbs turn to sugar in our bodies, triggering the pancreas to produce insulin, which instructs cells to mop up the toxic sugar in our blood to use immediately as fuel or to store as fat. But as the sugar levels fall, we feel tired and, yes, hungry.

We now eat more sugar in two weeks than our ancestors 300 years ago ate in an entire year, and this goes a long way towards explaining our so-called 'ageing diseases', such as diabetes. And guess what? We don't need to eat starchy carbs at all. The brain only needs the equivalent of a teaspoon of sugar a day to work properly, which we can get easily from a little fruit. But our body loves to burn carbs as fuel. If we put carbs in the tank, then our bodies simply won't bother to burn fat, happily leaving it around our tummies, hips and thighs, where we don't want it!

So what happens if we don't eat carbs? The body immediately starts to burn fat for energy. Not only that, it produces substances that mobilize fat and allow it to dissolve. If we stopped eating carbs, our calorie intake would automatically drop by about 1,000 calories. Also, you have seen how our bodies need insulin to absorb fat; that's why insulin is known as the 'fattening hormone'.

Insulin is the main regulator of fat, carbohydrate and protein metabolism. It regulates the synthesis of a molecule called glycogen – the form in which glucose is stored in muscle tissue and the liver – and stimulates the storage of fat, while inhibiting the release of that fat. It also stops your body producing cyclic adenosine monophosphate (AMP), which is a substance that stops your body storing fat. (Insulin also raises blood pressure, according to studies by endocrinologist Lewis Landsberg at the Harvard Medical School.)

In other words, if we don't eat carbs, we can eat 'fattening' foods without gaining weight *and* we'll feel less hungry. Stop the insulin surges and we will lose fat and stay thinner.

Sweet Poison

Starchy carbs are turned into the sugar maltose, which is converted into glucose in the body. So for instance, white bread, though it doesn't taste sweet like cakes and biscuits, literally turns to sugar in your system. And bread is seductively easy to eat. That bread that comes round before you even get your food in a restaurant, for example? Those breadsticks that are so quickly nibbled with a dip. We eat this kind of stuff not because we love it, but because it's there.

But if sugar is bad for us, is fruit unhealthy as so many trendy low-carb diet regimes claim? Of course not. It was a crazy idea to suggest that we should stay away from natural, unprocessed, healthy fruit with its phytonutrients and vitamins.

Science tells us not all sugars are created equal. Natural fructose, the type of sugar found in fruits, is 'good' sugar and is absorbed differently from glucose. Half the sugar in fructose is metabolized in the intestine and half by the liver, so none is left to circulate in the bloodstream. When you eat fruit, the body has to tear up the cells of the fruit to get at the sugar, which is also packaged with fibre, so there's no insulin surge. Studies show that fruit is safe to eat and does not raise blood sugar levels, even in diabetics.

Alcohol sugars, which are xylitol and sorbitol, are metabolized by the liver. Much of the sugar in alcohol isn't metabolized at all and simply passes out of the body in urine. Also, alcohol turns up your body thermostat, increasing the energy burn of other foods, which may be why those who have one or two drinks a day tend to be slimmer than teetotallers. This isn't a licence to go crazy, though, as alcohol has other harmful effects on the body, as well as hormonal effects, which we'll explain later.

Remember, all calories are not the same. Because of the

effects of insulin, calories eaten as carbs will cause you to gain more fat than calories eaten as protein and fat.

Passion for Protein

We need protein for the life, construction, replacement and repair of every cell in our body. It's the building block of our lives. Protein is also vital for the antibodies in our immune system, to regulate our temperature, and for energy in our muscles. Protein is a massively feel-good substance. Foods such as meat, fish, eggs and dairy can make us euphoric.

Remember, it takes three times as many calories to digest protein, compared to the calories it takes to digest carbs or fats. Yup, three times as many. So eat protein to fire up your metabolism.

What is Protein?

Protein is made up of amino acids, which are systems arranged in different combinations. Most amino acids can be made in our bodies, but there are eight vital amino acids we can only get in food:

- Isoleucine
- Leucine
- L-lysine
- Methionine
- Phenylalanine
- Threonine
- L-tryptophan
- Valine

Why do you need to know all that? Well, while we all know about vitamin and mineral supplements, few of us consider amino acid supplements, but these can be an important way to feel more youthful, happier and help you lose fat. That's because protein doesn't just build muscles, amino acids can serve as 'neurohormones', with dramatic effects on your mood and wellbeing.

Why Protein is Fantastic

- It blocks hunger pangs.
- It speeds up our metabolism.
- It takes more energy to digest than carbs or fats.
- It doesn't stimulate the fat hormone insulin.
- It is the most vital component of our body.

Fabulous Fat

Fat gets a really bad rap nowadays. It's blamed for just about every disease associated with ageing, plus, of course, it makes you fat. But is fat really evil? No. In fact fats, unlike carbs, are absolutely essential to our health. We can't produce our sex hormones without them, or absorb certain vital, health-giving, cancer-fighting vitamins, such as A, D, E and K. Cutting out fat might make us thin, but it will also make us malnourished and old.

However, you don't need fat wrapped up in processed food. Good fats, such as those found in nuts, avocados and butter, are delicious, nutritious, and it's actually hard to eat too much of them without lots of carbs. After all, you eat a lot less butter when there's no toast to spread it on. And what's more, fat without carbs isn't really absorbed by the body.

Fibre

We don't tend to think of fibre as a food group. It's the indigestible part of carbs, especially vegetables. So if it's not digested, it's useless, right? Wrong! Because fibre can absorb up to four times its weight in water, it gives us a feeling of fullness, as well as speeding food through the digestive process and trapping fat from food before it can be absorbed. It also reduces the amount of sugar in the blood, which may help protect us against diabetes. You'll lose weight – and fat – faster on a fibre-rich diet, and fibre is best found in fruit and vegetables.

Studies show that women who eat the most fruit and vegetables stay slimmer, keep more weight off after diets and are generally healthier, so eat as many different fruits and vegetables as you can, aiming for five to nine portions a day.

Water

The first rule for fat loss is – drink more water! If you really want to lose weight, drink two litres a day. Why?

- It curbs your appetite.
- It prevents water retention.
- It improves digestion.

But stop drinking water an hour before meals, and don't drink *with* meals. This means your stomach won't be full of water when you eat, diluting your vital digestive enzymes.

Ideally, drink your water ice cold, as your body uses calories to heat iced water to body temperature – energy it takes from your fat reserves.

While we are talking about drinks, avoid all sugary fizzy drinks, ideally for ever. Susie calls them the devil's drink. This includes supposedly healthy fruit juice. Even a can of a sweet fizzy drink each day for a month can alter our genes so that our muscles use sugar for energy instead of burning fat. This sugar is then processed by the liver and high doses can cause fat build-up in the liver, which can cause a type of cirrhosis. Diet fizzy drinks may be no better.

A 2013 study at Purdue University has linked diet fizzy drinks to obesity, diabetes and heart disease, just like their sugary counterparts. In fact, the study, which was actually a review of a whole host of previous studies, found that people who drank fizzy drinks with artificial sweeteners were even more likely to put on weight than those who drank the non-diet stuff.

Others studies found that diet soda doubled the risk of developing metabolic syndrome. Metabolic syndrome is the name for the combination of the poor blood sugar control known as insulin resistance, or full-blown diabetes, plus obesity, and high blood pressure. Women with metabolic syndrome have a waist of 35 inches (89 cm) or more. Metabolic syndrome affects an astounding one in four adults in the UK. The bad news is that it may raise your risk of heart disease and stroke. The good news is that it is preventable and reversible. So swap your fizzy drinks for water, eh?

One theory is that fake sweeteners confuse the body's ability to know how many calories it needs, leading to increased hunger and over-eating.

The Dr Sister Diet Rules

EAT MORE PROTEIN – Eat some kind of protein with every meal – think lean meat, poultry, eggs, yoghurt – and try to go as organic as possible to avoid the extra steroids, hormones and antibiotics usually found in non-organic meat.

CUT YOUR CARBS – Cut out all starchy and sugary carbs. Get your healthy carbs from fruit and vegetables. This doesn't mean you can never eat carbs again. Complex carbs, such as beans, whole grains and brown rice, can come back into your diet in controlled amounts when you are at your healthy weight. There is an exception at break-fast, when you can choose cereal to eat every other day. See the list on p. 238 for what you can't eat.

DRINK PLENTY OF WATER – two litres a day, ideally cold. Make sure you don't drink it with meals and leave it an hour before and after your meals.

EAT LOTS OF VEGETABLES – as much as you like. Not only are they full of fibre and nutrients, studies show women with a veg-heavy diet keep weight off best.

EAT FRUIT, BUT EAT IT SEPARATELY FROM MEALS – Eat it up to thirty minutes before meals or two hours after. The idea is not to have fat and sugar in the stomach at the same time. So no fruit for dessert, no fruit yogurt (which usually contains large amounts of sugar), and no fruit juice with breakfast. It's best to eat fruit mid-morning, at about 4 p.m., or a couple of hours after your evening meal.

EAT FAT, ESPECIALLY WITH VEGETABLES – The fibre stops you absorbing too much fat and the fat will help your body absorb vitamins from the vegetables.

WAIT TWENTY MINUTES AFTER A MEAL BEFORE YOU TAKE A SECOND HELPING – It takes that long for the receptors in the stomach and intestine to tell your brain you are full.

EAT ONLY WHEN YOU ARE HUNGRY – not because you are bored, tired, stressed or just to be polite. Your health comes first!

YOU CAN DRINK ALL THE TEA AND COFFEE YOU WANT – but with no sugar and no milk, except unsweetened rice or almond milk. Why? Milk contains the milk sugar lactose, while coffee contains caffeine. Together, caffeine and lactose are toxic for your liver, and we want your liver fully functioning for effective fat burning. Trust us, once you get used to it, good black high-quality coffee is actually nicer.

YOU CAN EAT BRAN AND OAT FLAKES, BUT ONLY FOR BREAKFAST – They are good for your digestion and you will burn these good carbs up throughout the day, plus they will give you that extra bit of energy. Try eating them every other day to drop a dress size. You can eat them with unsweetened almond or rice milk.

WE WANT YOU TO SUCCEED IN YOUR WEIGHT LOSS – but we know that you are only human, so while trying to lose weight you can allow yourself a maximum of two small glasses of wine, or a small (and we mean small) amount of spirits per day. If you do want to drink alcohol, we suggest drinking it an hour after your meal in the evening, or an hour before as an aperitif.

TRY TO EAT LITTLE AND OFTEN – to keep your metabolism revved. Eat every three hours, and avoid eating late in the evening to allow for effective overnight fat burning. Add exercise to the mix and watch the weight drop off.

CHEW AS SLOWLY AS YOU CAN

DRINK HERBAL TEAS – in the evening and throughout the day as they're a great thirst-quencher and can help you feel full in the evenings. We love Yogi Tea in Choco Aztec Spice, which actually tastes of chocolate, without any sugar or calories.

FORGET THE SCALES – Don't become obsessed with your scales. Your body shape and clothing size are more important than the numbers on your scales, and much less frustrating. As you follow our advice and exercise more, you will begin to build muscle. And remember, muscle weighs more than fat, therefore the figures on your scales can be misleading. Susie has a pair of jeans from when she was twenty. She holds onto them even though they are full of holes, and knows that when she can zip them up and breathe, she can relax.

Carb Foods You Can Have for Breakfast Only
while Dropping a Dress Size

- Oatmeal with water or rice or almond milk.
- Bran flakes or bran with rice or almond milk.

What You Can and Cannot Eat on this Programme

The Golden Rules of Dropping a Dress Size
Don't eat

Corn or anything made with cornstarch	Potatoes	Sugar
Balsamic vinegar (too much sugar)	Hummus, tahini, taramasalata	Honey
Cakes, biscuits and pastry – basically anything made of flour	Processed cheese	Pancakes
Nuts	Dried fruits and raisins	Bread
Fruit juice (most made from concentrate)	Margarine and spreads	Pasta
Processed meats, such as salami and bacon	Sweets/candy	Peas, lima beans, kidney beans, rice
Carbonated fizzy drinks/soda, even diet soda	Soya sauce	Milk

Eat as much as you like!

Natural, unprocessed meat	Eggs	Poultry	Unsweetened soya milk
Unsweetened natural yogurt	Butter	Goat's cheese	
Organic soya products (check ingredients, no sugar or starches)	Olive oil	Fish/shellfish	
Unprocessed cheese	Coconut oil	Coffee/tea	

(Note: try to go with organic as much as possible)

Vegetables you can eat as much of as you like

Artichokes	Celery	Leeks	Shallots
Asparagus	Courgettes	Lettuce	Spinach
Aubergine	Cucumbers	Mushrooms	Squash
Avocado	Endive	Onions	Turnips
Brussels sprouts	Garlic	Parsnips	Watercress
Cabbage	Green beans	Pumpkin	

Fruit, to be eaten separately from meals

Apples	Grapefruit	Oranges	Plums
Apricots	Grapes	Papaya	Prunes
Bananas (keep them for the days you exercise)	Mango	Peaches	Tangerines
Berries	Nectarines	Pears	Tomatoes
Cherries	Olives	Pineapple	Watermelon

Your Daily Diet Planner

These are just suggestions. Feel free to swap the meals around and remember, as long as you stick to the principles, you can make your own interesting meals to your own tastes. Pick foods you really enjoy, and add herbs and spices to make every meal a joy.

PLAN 1

Breakfast

Oat or bran flakes with fruit, yoghurt or rice or almond milk. Follow with a slice of turkey or chicken breast (unprocessed and organic if possible).

Mid-morning snack

Bunch of grapes and an apple.

Lunch

Goat's cheese salad, with olive oil and lemon dressing. Mix a bit of mustard into the dressing.

Afternoon snack

Chopped carrots, cucumbers and celery sticks with cheese slices. Try a mature cheddar with a spoonful of mustard to taste.

Dinner

Grilled salmon with crushed garlic and freshly ground black pepper, asparagus, mushrooms and broccoli. Grill the vegetables with coconut or olive oil and sprinkle some Parmesan shavings on top.

After dinner

Wine (if you want it) and some olives.

PLAN 2

Breakfast

Smoked salmon and scrambled eggs garnished with parsley and freshly ground black pepper.

Mid-morning snack

Pineapple slice, fresh blueberries, raspberries and pomegranates.

Lunch

Vegetable soup, with a side salad of grilled vegetables on lettuce with grated cheese on top. Olive oil and lemon dressing.

Afternoon snack

Cucumber and celery sticks with low-fat cream cheese and olives.

Dinner

Roast organic chicken with roasted garlic and shallots, served with buttered spinach and/or mixed vegetables.

After dinner

A glass of wine and/or a sliced apple and pear.

PLAN 3

Breakfast

Poached eggs with mushrooms and tomatoes. (OK– tomatoes are a fruit, but they are allowed.)

Mid-morning snack

Some Greek yoghurt.

Lunch

A large mixed salad with prawns or chicken.

Afternoon snack

Fresh fruit salad.

Dinner

Tuna steak with fresh pesto sauce (make sure it's sugar free) and grilled or stir-fried vegetables.

After dinner

Grapes or watermelon.

PLAN 4

Breakfast

Oatmeal or bran flakes with unsweetened rice or almond milk.

Mid-morning snack

Unsweetened Greek yogurt or fruit.

Lunch

Roast beef, chicken or turkey salad.

Afternoon snack

Slices of cheese with celery and carrot sticks.

Dinner

Fish/chicken and vegetable curry.

After dinner

Glass of wine or herbal tea, grilled artichokes or olives.

PLAN 5

Breakfast

Cheese omelette with fresh herbs.

Mid-morning snack

Unsweetened Greek yogurt or fruit.

Lunch

A large green salad with avocado and prawns.

Afternoon snack

Freshly sliced watermelon and pineapple.

Dinner

Organic steak with garlic butter, onions and a selection of vegetables.

After dinner

Strawberries.

It Worked for Me!

Emma Parson, fifty-five, a marketing manager, says, 'Since hitting the menopause two years ago, I'd gained nearly a stone, mostly around my middle, and working out and cutting calories just wasn't working any more.

'I tried the Dr Sister diet and, to my amazement, lost 4 lbs in the first week, while eating steak, cheese, fruit and butter. It was so easy. I particularly loved that I could eat fruit, as I'd tried the Dukan and Atkins diets and hated not being able to snack on fruit. I didn't think it was healthy to cut it out, plus fruit is crunchy, convenient when you are out and really satisfies a sweet tooth.

'Also, on this diet I was never hungry, cold or tired, as I was when trying to do intermittent fasting. It's a diet you can eat out on, and even drink wine on. It's perfect for my lifestyle. I've lost 8 lbs in three weeks and can see my waist again.'

Remember, once you drop down to your ideal weight, just follow the suggestions in our 'Eat Yourself Young' and 'Metabolism' chapters and enjoy! You can always dip in and out of the drop-a-dress-size diet if you want to lose a few pounds gained on holiday, but don't let yourself get too thin. It's not good for your hormones or the way you look, plus being too thin is terribly ageing for the skin.

Take Control!

- Not all calories are created equal.
- Muscle weighs more than fat, so don't worry about the scales.
- Cut out carbs except for breakfast.
- Timing is everything.
- Eat fruit separately.

'Never eat more than you can lift.'
  Miss Piggy

25 Be-Youthful Daily Reminders

Get Some Attitude!

1. Ageing is not just something that happens to us, it's controlled by the choices we make and the lifestyles we lead. This means we can change our age destiny.
2. Hang out with younger people. It could help you live longer, and weddings are more fun than funerals!
3. Stop telling people your age – 'old enough' is a perfectly good answer.
4. Stop whining about your age and ailments and do something positive instead. Encourage your friends to do the same.
5. Never think there's anything you can't do because you are 'too old'. Do stuff you love, that makes you feel passionate, happy and alive. Studies show that a smile takes as many years off your face as a surgical facelift.

Eat Yourself Young

6. Swap processed, hydrogenated fats for olive oil, nuts and nut oils, avocado and coconut oil.
7. Try to go twelve hours overnight without eating or drinking anything except water as often as you can.
8. Go sixteen hours without eating overnight once or twice a week, providing you can still sleep well.
9. To lose weight you need to cut insulin levels, so cut out sweet and starchy carbs. Insulin is the fattening hormone.
10. Eat metabolism-boosting foods, especially protein, at every meal.
11. Drink two litres of water a day – ideally chilled.
12. When you want to snack, make raw nuts or berries your number one choice.
13. Use tricks to cut your portion size – choose smaller, blue plates.

Anti-Age Your Lifestyle

14. Exercise most days. It can add seven years to your life expectancy. Try yoga, Pilates or walking or running outdoors, and mix it up a bit.
15. Take up meditation of some kind. Prayer counts, too.

16. Sleep more and better. Aim for at least seven hours a night, ideally more.
17. Spend more time with good, positive, friends. Fun is fabulously de-stressing, and a good network of friends may make you live longer.
18. Change what you realistically can, and learn to cope with what you can't.
19. Take a break from your desk every twenty minutes.
20. Stand tall. Good posture can strengthen your core, protect your back, take years off your appearance and even change your hormones.

Give Yourself Some Love

21. An orgasm is an orgasm no matter how you get it – and it's the best de-stresser ever.
22. If you believe you look younger, other people will perceive you as younger! Book that hair appointment now. Buy those ah-maz-ing shoes.
23. Think about taking hormones when you hit the menopause for an improved quality of life and a younger face and body.
24. Adopt a positive attitude. It's almost impossible to smile and worry at the same time. Go on, try it!
25. Take control. Your chronological age has never mattered less. You can achieve anything you put your mind to.